SOAP
for
Obstetrics and Gynecology

Look for other books in this series!

SOAP
for
Obstetrics and Gynecology

Peter S. Uzelac, MD, FACOG
Assistant Professor
Department of Obstetrics and Gynecology
University of Southern California Keck School of Medicine
Los Angeles, California

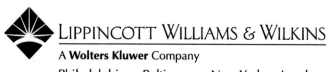

LIPPINCOTT WILLIAMS & WILKINS
A **Wolters Kluwer** Company
Philadelphia · Baltimore · New York · London
Buenos Aires · Hong Kong · Sydney · Tokyo

351 West Camden Street
Baltimore, Maryland 21201-2436 USA

530 Walnut Street
Philadelphia, Pennsylvania 19106-3621 USA

Printed in the United States of America

Library of Congress Cataloging-in-Publication Data

Uzelac, Peter S.
    SOAP for obstetrics and gynecology / Peter S. Uzelac.
    p. ; cm.
    Includes index.
    ISBN 978-1-4051-0435-7 (pbk.)
    ISBN 1-4051-0435-X (pbk.)
    1. Obstetrics—Handbooks, manuals, etc. 2. Gynecology—Handbooks,
manuals, etc. [DNLM: 1. Genital Diseases, Female—Handbooks. 2. Obstetrics—
Handbooks. 3. Pregnancy Complications—Handbooks. WP 39 U99s 2005]
    I. Title.

RG110.U985 2005
618—dc22   2004005831

A catalogue record for this title is available from the British Library

Editor: Donna Balado
Managing Editor: Kathleen Scogna
Marketing Manager: Emilie Linkins

To purchase additional copies of this book call our customer service department at (800) 638-3030 or fax orders to (301) 824-7390. International customers should call (301) 714-2324.

Visit Lippincott Williams & Wilkins on the Internet: http://www.lww.com. Lippincott Williams & Wilkins customer service representatives are available from 8:30 am to 6:00 pm, EST, Monday through Friday, for telephone access.

12 13 14

To my wife, Alina

Iubirea, prietena, partenera mea în această călătorie minunat

Contents

To the Reader

Like most medical students, I started my ward experience head down and running, eager to finally make contact with real patients. What I found was a confusing world, completely different from anything I had known during the first two years of medical school. New language, foreign abbreviations and residents too busy to set my bearings straight: Where would I begin?

Pocket textbooks, offering medical knowledge in a convenient and portable package, seemed to be the logical solution. Unfortunately, I found myself spending valuable time sifting through large amounts of text, often not finding the answer to my question, and in the process, missing out on teaching points during rounds!

I designed the SOAP series to provide medical students and house staff with pocket manuals that truly serve their intended purpose: quick accessibility to the most practical clinical information in a user-friendly format. At the inception of this project, I envisioned all of the benefits the SOAP format would bring to the reader:

- Learning through this model reinforces a thought process that is already familiar to students and residents, facilitating easier long-term retention.

- SOAP promotes good communication between physicians and facilitates the teaching/learning process.

- SOAP puts the emphasis back on the patient's clinical problem and not the diagnosis.

- In the age of managed care, SOAP meets the challenge of providing efficiency while maintaining quality.

- As sound medical-legal practice gains attention in physician training, SOAP emphasizes adherence to a documentation style that leaves little room for potential misinterpretation.

Rather than attempting to summarize the contents of a thousand-page textbook into a miniature form, the SOAP series focuses exclusively on guidance through patient encounters. In a typical use, "finding out where to start" or "refreshing your memory" with SOAP books should be possible in less than a minute. Subjects are always confined to two pages and the most important points have been highlighted. Topics have been limited to those problems you will most commonly encounter repeatedly during your training and contents are grouped according to the hospital or clinic setting. Facts and figures that are not particularly helpful to surviving life on the wards, such as demographics, pathophysiology and busy tables and graphs have purposely been omitted (such details are much better studied in a quiet environment using large and comprehensive texts).

Congratulations on your achievements thus far and I wish you a highly successful medical career!

Peter S. Uzelac, MD, FACOG

Acknowledgments

I would foremost like to thank my own teachers, the physicians who have taught me their art and instilled in me the desire to pass on this knowledge to others. Special appreciation to Beverly Copland for her enthusiasm and motivation from this project's infancy, Selene Steneck for her patience and persistence in keeping this project on track, and all of the SOAP authors for their hard work and commitment to making this series a success.

Contributor

Alina Uzelac, D.O.
Resident in Radiology
University of Southern California
Los Angeles, California

Reviewers

SoHyun Boo
Class of 2005
West Virginia University School of Medicine
Morgantown, West Virginia

Melanie Endres
Class of 2005
UMDNJ—Robert Wood Johnson School of Medicine
New Brunswick, New Jersey

Deleshia Kinney, MAT
Class of 2005
Southern Illinois University School of Medicine
Springfield, Illinois

C. Anne Morrison
Class of 2005
Medical University of South Carolina
Charleston, South Carolina

Arne Olsen
Class of 2004
Medical College of Wisconsin
Milwaukee, Wisconsin

Leontine Narcisse
Class of 2005
Albert Einstein College of Medicine
Bronx, New York

Abbreviations

A-a gradient	alveolar-to-arterial gradient
ABG	arterial blood gas
AC	abdominal circumference
ADA	American Diabetic Association
AFI	amniotic fluid index
AFP	alpha-fetoprotein
Alt	alternative regimen
AP testing	antepartum testing
APS	antiphospholipid syndrome
ARDS	adult respiratory distress syndrome
AUB	abnormal uterine bleeding
β-hCG	beta human chorionic gonadotropin
bid	*bis in die* (twice daily)
BMD	bone mineral density
BMI	body mass index
BP	blood pressure
BPM	beats per minute
BPP	biophysical profile
BV	bacterial vaginosis
CA	cancer
CA125	cancer antigen 125 test
CBC	complete blood count
CHF	congestive heart failure
CHTN	chronic hypertension
CMP	comprehensive metabolic panel
CMT	cervical motion tenderness
CMV	cytomegalovirus
CPP	chronic pelvic pain
CRF	chronic renal failure
C/S	cesarean section
CST	contraction stress test
CT	computed tomography
CVAT	costovertebral angle tenderness
CXR	chest x-ray
DBP	diastolic blood pressure
D&C	dilation and curettage
DES	diethylstilbestrol
DEXA	dual-energy x-ray absorptiometry
DHEAS	dehydroepiandrosterone sulfate
DM	diabetes mellitus
DNA	deoxyribonucleic acid
DUB	dysfunctional uterine bleeding
DVT	deep vein thrombosis
EBL	estimated blood loss
EC	emergency contraception
ECG	electrocardiogram
EDC	estimated date of confinement

EFW	estimated fetal weight
EGA	estimated gestational age
EMB	endometrial biopsy
FFN	fetal fibronectin
FH	fundal height
FHRT	fetal heart rate tracing
FM	fetal movement
FNA	fine-needle aspiration
FSH	follicle-stimulating hormone
FTA-ABS	fluorescent treponemal antibody absorption
GBS	group B streptococcus
GCT	glucose challenge test
GDM	gestational diabetes mellitus
GI	gastrointestinal
GS	gestational sac
GSUI	genuine stress urinary incontinence
GTD	gestational trophoblastic disease
GTT	glucose tolerance test
GU	genitourinary
H/A	headache
Hb	hemoglobin
HBsAg	hepatitis B surface antigen
HCG	human chorionic gonadotropin
Hct	hematocrit
HEENT	head, ears, eyes, nose, and throat
HELLP	hemolysis, elevated liver enzymes, low platelets
HIV	human immunodeficiency virus
HPV	human papilloma virus
hr(s)	hour(s)
HRT	hormone replacement therapy
HSV	herpes simplex virus
ICSI	intracytoplasmic sperm injection
IM	intramuscular
IMM	intramyometrial
I/O	input and output
IUD	intrauterine device
IUGR	intrauterine growth restriction
IUI	intrauterine insemination
IUP	intrauterine pregnancy
IV	intravenous
IVF	in-vitro fertilization
KOH	potassium hydroxide
LAC	lupus anticoagulant
lb	pound
L&D	labor and delivery
LFT	liver function test
LH	luteinizing hormone
LMP	last menstrual period
L:S	lecithin/syphingomyelin ratio
MCV	mean corpuscular volume

MgSO$_4$	magnesium sulfate
MI	myocardial infarction
MOM	multiples of the mean
MPA	medroxyprogesterone acetate
MRI	magnetic resonance imaging
MSAFP	maternal serum alpha-fetoprotein
MVA	manual vacuum aspiration
NPH	neutral protamine Hagedorn insulin
NPO	*nulla per os* (nothing by mouth)
NS	normal saline
NSAID	nonsteroidal anti-inflammatory drug
NST	nonstress test
NTD	neural tube defect
N/V	nausea and vomiting
NVP	nausea and vomiting of pregnancy
OC	oral contraceptive
PAP	Papanicolaou smear
PCOS	polycystic ovary syndrome
PE	physical exam
PEFR	peak expiratory flow rate
PGBS	post-glucose blood sugar
PID	pelvic inflammatory disease
PIH	pregnancy-induced hypertension
PMH	past medical history
PMS	premenstrual syndrome
PO	*per os* (by mouth)
POC	products of conception
POD	postoperative day
PPH	postpartum hemorrhage
PPROM	preterm premature spontaneous rupture of membranes
PPTL	postpartum tubal ligation
PR	per rectum
PRN	*pro re nata* (as needed)
PROM	premature spontaneous rupture of membranes
PSH	past surgical history
Pt(s)	patient(s)
PT	prothrobin time
PTB	preterm birth
PTL	preterm labor
PTT	partial thromboplastin time
PTU	propylthiouracil
PUBS	percutaneous umbilical blood sampling
PUD	peptic ulcer disease
q	*quodque* (every)
qd	*quaque die* (once daily)
qh	*quaque hora* (every hour)
qid	*quater in die* (four times daily)
RBCs	red blood cells
Rec	recommended regimen
RDA	recommended daily allowance

RDS	respiratory distress syndrome
ROM	rupture of membranes
ROS	review of systems
RPL	recurrent pregnancy loss
RPR	rapid plasma reagin
RUQ	right upper quadrant
SAB	spontaneous abortion
SBP	systolic blood pressure
SERM	selective estrogen receptor modulator
SLE	systemic lupus erythematosus
SQ	subcutaneous
SSRI	selective serotonin reuptake inhibitor
STD	sexually transmitted disease
tid	*ter in die* (thrice daily)
TOA	tubo-ovarian abscess
TOL	trial of labor
TSH	thyroid-stimulating hormone
TSS	toxic shock syndrome
U/A	urinalysis
UC	uterine contraction
URI	upper respiratory tract infection
U/S	ultrasound
UTI	urinary tract infection
UVJ	urethral-vesicular junction
VS	vital signs
WBCs	white blood cells
wks	weeks
y/o	years old

Normal Lab Values

Blood, Serum, Plasma

Albumin	3.9–5.0 g/dL
Alkaline Phosphatase	38–126 IU/L
Aminotransferase, alanine (ALT, SGPT)	0–35 U/L
Aminotransferase, aspartate (AST, SGOT)	0–35 U/L
Ammonia	40–80 μg/dL
Amylase	0–130 IU/L
Bicarbonate	23–28 meq/L
Bilirubin	
Total	0.3–1.2 mg/dL
Direct	0–0.4 mg/dL
Calcium	8.4–10.5 mg/dL
Carbon dioxide	23–28 meq/L
Chloride	98–106 meq/L
Cholesterol, total	150–199 mg/dL (desirable)
Cholesterol, low-density lipoprotein (LDL)	≤ 130 mg/dL (desirable)
Cholesterol, high-density lipoprotein (HDL)	≥ 40 mg/dL (desirable)
Creatinine	0.7–1.4 mg/dL
Ferritin	6–186 ng/mL
Fibrinogen	200–400 mg/dL
Glucose	70–110 mg/dL
Iron	37–170 μg/dL
Iron binding capacity	250–460 μg/dL
Lactate dehydrogenase	60–100 IU/L
Lipase	< 95 U/L
Magnesium	1.5–2.0 mEq/L
Osmolality	275–295 mosm/kg
Phosphorus	2.5–4.5 mg/dL
Potassium	3.5–5.3 mEq/L
Protein, Total	6.3–8.2 g/dL
Sodium	136–145 meq/L
Triglycerides	< 250 mg/dL (desirable)
Urea nitrogen	5–25 mg/dL
Uric acid	2.5–7.5 mg/dL

Endocrine

Adrenocorticotropin hormone (ACTH)

6:00 AM	9–90 pg/mL	2–11 pmol/L
6:00 PM	< 60 pg/mL	< 11 pmol/L

Androstenedione   85–275 ng/dL   3.0–9.6 nmol/L

Cortisol

8:00 AM	8–20 μg/dL	221–552 nmol/L
5:00 PM	3–13 μg/dL	83–359 nmol/L
10:00 PM	< 50% AM value	< 50% AM value

Dehydroepiandrosterone sulfate   30–379 μg/dL   0.8–10.2 μmol/L

Estradiol

Follicular phase	20–150 pg/mL	73–550 pmol/L
Midcycle	150–750 pg/mL	550–2750 pmol/L
Luteal phase	30–450 pg/mL	100–1650 pmol/L
Postmenopausal	< 20 pg/mL	< 73 pmol/L

Follicle-stimulating hormone (FSH)

Reproductive age	5–30 mIU/mL	5–30 U/L
Postmenopausal	> 35 mU/mL	> 35 U/L

Glucose, fasting   70–110 mg/dL

Glucose Challenge Test, 1 hour/50 g   < 140 mg/dL (normal)

Glucose Tolerance Test, 3 hour/100 g   < 95/180/155/140 mg/dL (normal)

17-Hydroxyprogesterone   100–300 ng/mL   3–9 nmol/L

Insulin, fasting   5–20 mIU/L   35–180 pmol/L

Luteinizing hormone (LH)

Reproductive age	5–22 mIU/mL	5–22 IU/L

Progesterone

Follicular phase	< 3 ng/mL	< 9.5 nmol/L
Luteal phase	5–30 ng/mL	16–95 nmol/L

Prolactin   3.8–23.2 ng/mL   3.8–23.2 μg/L

Testosterone

Free	100–200 pg/dL	35–700 pmol/L
Total	20–75 ng/dL	0.7–2.6 nmol/L

Thyroid-stimulating hormone (TSH)   0.35–6.7 μU/mL   0.35–6.7 mU/L

Thyroxine (T4)

Free	0.9–2.4 ng/dL	12–31 pmol/L
Total	5–12 μg/dL	71–142 nmol/L

Triiodothyronine (T3)

Free	0.13–0.55 ng/dL	2.0–8.5 pmol/L
Total	80–220 ng/dL	71–142 nmol/L

Hematology and Coagulation

Activated partial thromboplastin time (APTT)	25–35 seconds
Bleeding time	< 10 minutes
D-Dimer	< 0.25 mg/L
Hematocrit	35–47%
Hemoglobin	11.7–15.7 g/dL
Leukocyte count	4–11 K/μL
Poly	42–73%
Mono	2–11%
Lymph	12–40%
Eos	0–7%
Baso	0–2%
Bands	0–11%
Mean corpuscular hemoglobin (MCH)	28–32 pg
Mean corpuscular hemoglobin concentration (MCHC)	32–36 g/dL
Mean corpuscular volume (MCV)	80–100 fL
Platelet count	150–350 K/μL
Prothrombin time (PT)	11–13 seconds
PT-INR	0.89–1.11 INR
Red Blood Cells	3.8–5.2 MIL/μL
Red Cell Distribution of Width (RDW)	11.5–14.6%

I

Obstetrics Clinic

S **Is the pt sure about the date of her last menstrual period (LMP)?**
LMP is customarily used to establish the estimated gestational age (EGA) and
estimated date of confinement (EDC) (or "due date").

- An accurate EGA/EDC is the single most important piece of information to be
known about a pregnancy.

An *unsure* LMP warrants an ultrasound examination to establish EGA/EDC.
- A history of irregular periods or hormonal contraception use before conception
may also warrant an U/S, especially if your physical examination of the uterus is
inconsistent with proposed dates (see below).
- Methods to "date" a pregnancy of unknown age (e.g., ultrasound, physical exam)
become progressively more inaccurate as the pregnancy advances.

- Therefore, it is crucial to establish the EGA/EDC early in pregnancy.

Review obstetric history
Identify any obstetric problems that may recur with current pregnancy.
Pts with previous pregnancies affected by NTDs should be on folate 4 mg/day.

Perform ROS and obtain PMH
Elicit a history of any potential medical problems complicating pregnancy.

Obtain PSH
Pts with previous C/S should be counseled regarding delivery options for current
pregnancy:
                - Trial of labor   - Repeat C/S

Obtain Social history
Alcohol, tobacco, and substance use should be identified and counseled appropriately.

Obtain Family history
Pts with a family history of congenital anomalies, mental retardation, or metabolic
diseases should be identified and referred for prenatal diagnosis (see Second Trimester
Visit p. 4).

Does the pt have any high-risk factors for gestational diabetes mellitus (GDM)?
GDM is a major contributor to morbidity in pregnancy (see GDM p. 18).
Identifying potentially affected individuals early can minimize complications.
The presence of any of the following high-risk factors warrants first trimester screening
for GDM:
                - History of glucose intolerance   - First-degree relative with DM
                - Adverse obstetric outcomes usually associated with GDM

Does the pt have any risk factors for antiphospholipid syndrome (APS)?
The presence of any of the following warrants a work-up for APS (see APS p. 12):
                - History of recurrent abortion (3 or more first trimester losses) or a single
                  second or third trimester fetal loss
                - Severe preeclampsia < 34 wks
                - Severe fetal growth restriction
                - History of thrombosis

O **Confirm a positive pregnancy test (β-hCG)**
Pregnancy can be confirmed with either a qualitative β-hCG (test is performed with a
urine specimen and reported as positive or negative) or a quantitative β-hCG (test is
performed with a blood sample and reported as a numeric value).

Is the EGA 10 wks or older?
If so, attempt to elicit fetal heart tones by doppler monitor.
Establishing heart tones helps confirm the EGA.

Perform PE
Careful attention should be paid to thyroid, cardiac, and pulmonary systems, which are
  most commonly associated with serious medical complications in pregnancy.
Uterine size should be confirmed to be consistent with EGA.
  • If your physical examination of the uterus is inconsistent with EGA, obtain U/S.

Is the pt obese? (BMI > 30)
Obese pts have a higher risk of glucose intolerance and should also be tested for GDM
  in first trimester.
Caloric requirements during pregnancy should be limited (total weight gain = 30 lbs).

Is glycosuria present on the office urine dip?
Some glycosuria is expected (caused by decreased tubular reabsorption), but a positive
  result on a second voided fasting urine warrants first trimester testing for GDM.

A   **Intrauterine pregnancy (IUP) at 8 wks**
Differential diagnosis of an early IUP includes any form of abnormal pregnancy:
         - Ectopic pregnancy   - Missed abortion   - Molar pregnancy

P   **Perform or schedule U/S if EGA is unclear**
Indications include unsure LMP or discrepancy on PE.

Draw the "prenatal" labs:
Blood group, Rh status, and antibody screen, CBC, Rubella, RPR, and HBsAg
Perform Pap smear and gonococcus/chlamydia cultures.
MSAFP if between 15 to 20 wks at initial visit (see Second Trimester Visit p. 4)

Prescribe prenatal vitamins and iron supplementation
Folate is the most important element for its association with prevention of NTDs
  (recommended intake 0.4 mg/day).
  • Ideally, pts should be taking some source of folate supplementation for 3 months
    before conception.
Iron supplementation helps the mother maintain iron stores in the face of increased
  requirement during pregnancy.

Instruct and educate pt about common questions and complaints
Diet, sleep, bowel habits, exercise, bathing, clothing, recreation, and travel
  • Up to 30% of all pts will experience vaginal spotting during first trimester.

Schedule next appointment
For an uncomplicated pregnancy, see pt every 4 wks in first trimester.

Consider referral to high-risk clinic
A pt with any medical problems should always be considered to receive care or
  consultation from a high-risk clinic.

S **If the pt was previously suffering from symptoms associated with the first trimester, are these resolving?**

Nausea and vomiting of pregnancy, fatigue, and associated symptoms should usually be declining by the second trimester.

Any persistent symptoms mandate workup for etiology.

Does the pt have any new complaints?

As the uterus enlarges, some women start to experience discomfort from the stretching of pelvic ligaments.

- "Round ligament pain" is a common diagnosis during the second trimester.

Preterm UCs should be worked up.

Does the pt belong to an ethnic group that has a high risk for specific genetic disorders?

Consider screening tests in the following populations:

- Eastern European (Ashkenazi) Jewish
  - Tay-Sachs and Canavan disease
- Cajun and French-Canadian
  - Tay-Sachs
- Caucasian
  - Cystic fibrosis

O **Check blood pressure**

Maternal blood pressure falls for the first 24 wks of pregnancy and then returns to normal values by term, secondary to relaxation effect of progesterone on smooth muscle.

- Diastolic pressure falls greater than systolic, widening pulse pressure.

Check urine dip for glucose and protein

Glucose > 1+ (> 100 mg/dL) may require earlier screening for GDM.

Proteinuria ≥ 2+ (≥ 100 mg/dL) requires urine analysis for infection and close observation of BP for preeclampsia.

Confirm appropriate maternal weight gain

Total weight gain for pregnancy should be about 30 lbs.

- 5 lbs should be gained in the first trimester.
- 1/2 to 1 lb/week should be gained for the remainder of pregnancy.
  - <10 lb weight gain by 20 wks should prompt a nutritional review.

Elicit fetal heart tones with doppler

This confirms ongoing viability of pregnancy.

Measure fundal height (FH)

This helps confirm ongoing fetal growth.

- If EGA < 20 wks, a rough estimate can be made by palpation.
- If EGA > 20 wks, assess by measuring fundal height in centimeters.

Measurement of FH in centimeters should equal EGA in wks.

A IUP at 17 wks

P **Offer the expanded MSAFP test (a.k.a. "triple screen")**
The expanded MSAFP test is a screening test used to detect NTDs and trisomies 18 and
   21 in the general population.
- This test is available to *all* pregnant pts and is performed between 15 to 20 wks.
- Detects 90% of NTDs and 60% of trisomies 18 and 21.
- The following markers are measured in maternal serum:
  - Alpha-fetoprotein (MSAFP)
  - hCG
  - Estriol

NTD screening uses the MSAFP value (alone).
- Algorithms are used that adjust for maternal weight and EGA.
- Results are reported as MOM.
  - MSAFP values > 2.5 MOM are considered a positive screen and require further
    workup in the form of an amniocentesis and U/S (see more below).

MSAFP, hCG, and estriol are analyzed for risk of trisomies 18 and 21 (Down
   syndrome).
- Results vary by maternal age, with older women having a higher screen positive
  rate.
  - *Low* MSAFP (< 0.7 MOM) and *low* estriol coupled with *elevated* hCG is
    considered a positive screen for trisomy 21 and warrants an amniocentesis and
    U/S for further evaluation.
  - A low value for all three analytes is considered a positive screen for trisomy 18.

Offer prenatal diagnosis to all pts with an indication
Prenatal diagnosis is a process by which pts at high risk for genetic abnormalities are
   worked up.
Process consists of genetic counseling followed by one or more of the following tests:
- Triple screen (as described above)
- Ultrasound
- Amniocentesis
  - Amniotic fluid is obtained by transabdominal needle aspiration under U/S
    guidance.
  - Collected fluid (with its amniotic cells) may be analyzed for:
    - Chromosomes (for detection of trisomies)
    - Acetylcholinesterse and alpha-fetoprotein (both of which are elevated with
      NTDs)
    - Specific genetic defects

Pts with the following history should be offered prenatal diagnosis:
- Pts with a positive *screen* for either an NTD or trisomy
- Birth defects in previous pregnancies
- Genetic disorders
- Exposure to teratogens
- Suspected fetal anomalies
- Pregestational diabetes mellitus
- Patients who are ≥ 35 y/o by their EDC

   - Women of advanced reproductive age have a higher risk for Down syndrome
     and therefore require a test that is more sensitive than the triple screen.

Schedule next appointment
For an uncomplicated pregnancy, see patient every 2 to 4 wks between 13 and 36 wks.

S   Is the fetus moving?

Any report of decreased fetal movement can signal fetal intolerance to the intrauterine environment and mandates some sort of antepartum testing (see below).

Is the pt experiencing any uterine contractions?

Any contractions < 35 wks should have workup for PTL (see PTL p. 50).

Pts with contractions > 35 wks should have cervical exam to assess dilatation.

Does the pt have any symptoms of preeclampsia?

New-onset visual complaints, headaches, or abdominal pain should raise suspicion for preeclampsia, and blood pressure should be examined closely.

O   Check blood pressure

BP should be carefully monitored in third trimester for preeclampsia.

- Because BP is usually decreased in pregnancy, even a high normal value should be rechecked.

Check urine dip for protein

Proteinuria ≥ 2+ (≥ 100 mg/dL) requires urine analysis for infection and close observation of BP for preeclampsia.

Confirm appropriate maternal weight gain

1/2 to 1 lb/week should be gained throughout third trimester.

- Excessive weight gain may signal excessive fluid retention, which can be associated with PIH.

Elicit fetal heart tones with doppler

Doppler heart tones confirm ongoing viability of pregnancy.

Measure fundal height (FH)

This helps confirm ongoing fetal growth.
- After 20 wks, the FH in centimeters should equal the estimated gestational age in wks.

Order 1-hr post glucose blood sugar (PGBS)

At 24 to 28 wks, pt should have a diabetes screen performed with a 1-hr PGBS.
- Pts ingest a 50-g load of glucose (in the form of a flavored drink).
- Serum glucose levels are measured 1 hour later.

Values above 140 mg/dL are abnormal and require further evaluation (see GDM p. 18).

Repeat CBC and RPR at 24 to 28 wks
Administer anti-D immune globulin to eligible pts at 28 wks

Anti-D immune globulin is administered at around 28 wks to pts who are Rh negative with no antibodies currently in serum (see Isoimmunization p. 24).

A   IUP at 28 wks

P   Instruct pt on potential experiences or problems

All pts should be instructed to go to L&D immediately for evaluation of any symptoms
   of labor or rupture of membranes.
Decreased fetal movement (FM) can be a sign of fetal morbidity and requires
   evaluation (see AP testing below).

Schedule follow-up visit

Visits every 2 to 3 wks until 36 wks
Visits every week from 37 wks until delivery

Check a GBS culture at 35 to 37 wks

Group B streptococcus (GBS) can be found as part of the normal flora around the
   vaginal introitus and rectal area of some women.
Carriers may vertically transmit GBS to the neonate during labor and delivery, where it
   can cause septicemia, pneumonia, or menigitis during the first week of life.
   - Such disease is known as early-onset GBS infection (to distinguish it from
      late-onset GBS infection, which is nosocomial or community-acquired).
Administration of antibiotics to GBS carriers during labor helps prevent early-onset
   disease.
   - Penicillin 5 million units IV load then 2.5 million units IV q 4 hrs until delivery
      (Rec)
   - Clindamycin 900 mg IV q 8 hrs until delivery (Alt)

Consider antepartum (AP) testing

High-risk pregnancies have an increased amount of fetal morbidity and mortality.
   - AP testing provides an objective way to assess fetal well-being during third
      trimester of pregnancy.
Currently accepted *indications for AP testing* include the following:
   - Fetal
      - Decreased FM, postdates (EGA > 40 wks), PIH, IUGR, oligohydramnios,
         polyhydramnios, multiple gestations, previous fetal demise
   - Maternal
      - CHTN, DM, SLE, CRF, APS, uncontrolled hyperthyroidism,
         hemoglobinopathies, cyanotic heart disease
The most popular method of AP testing is the combination of NST and AFI.
   - The NST consists of monitoring the fetal heart rate for a 20-minute period.
      - A reactive NST, defined as two episodes of an increase in the fetal heart rate of
         at least 15 BPM for at least 15 seconds, is a reassuring sign of fetal well-being.
      - Absent accelerations (nonreactive NST) requires further evaluation (see
         below).
   - The AFI is an ultrasonographic measurement of the amount of amniotic fluid.
      - Normal AFI is 5 to 25 cm
Other methods of AP testing are the contraction stress test (CST) and the biophysical
   profile (BPP).
   - The CST consists of monitoring the fetal heart rate in the presence of induced
      contractions.
      - This assesses how the fetus responds to an environment of stress (contractions).
   - The BPP is an assessment of fetal well-being based on five objective criteria:
      - NST, AFI, FM, tone, and breathing (assessed by U/S)
      - Each parameter is scored with a 0 or 2 (maximum score 10).
      - Subsequent management is based on score.

S **How is the pt doing since delivery?**

This open-ended question gives the pt an opportunity to raise any concerns she may be having.

- Review delivery before beginning the conversation, noting any complications.
- This is an appropriate time to screen for *postpartum depression* or *psychosis*.

Is the pt breastfeeding?

Inquire about any problems.

Is the pt having any abnormal bleeding? Fevers?

Lochia usually stops by the third postpartum week but can be present in a minority of women at the time of the postpartum check (see below).

If the pt had a C/S, how is the wound healing?

Occasionally, pts complain about a tingling or burning sensation around the wound, which is the result of cut nerves.

Is the pt experiencing normal voiding and bowel movements?

Postpartum urge and stress incontinence usually improve with time.
Postpartum constipation can be a source of discomfort.

Has pt resumed sexual intercourse?

Atrophic vaginitis, changes in libido, fatigue, and general perineal discomfort can affect the resumption of relations in the postpartum period.

How is the pt's diet?

Encourage plenty of fluids for sufficient milk production and as prophylaxis or treatment for constipation.

What are the pt's plans for future pregnancies?

Knowing the future childbearing plans provides the basis for selecting an appropriate contraceptive.

O **Perform physical examination**

Breasts
- Check for masses, engorgement, or signs of infection.

C/S wound should be dry, closed, and usually pink in color.

Pelvic
- External genitalia
  - ◆ Verify healing of any episiotomy or laceration from delivery.
  - ◆ Verify external genitalia are anatomically correct.
- Cervix
  - ◆ Observe for any lesions.
  - ◆ Review last Pap and repeat if warranted.
    - Previously abnormal Paps should have a workup completed postpartum.
- Uterus
  - ◆ Verify that uterus is involuted and non-tender.
  - ◆ Verify that postpartum discharge from uterus (lochia) is absent or sparse.
  - ◆ There are three stages to lochia:
    - Lochia rubra: 3 to 4 days, mostly bloody and thick
    - Lochia serosa: 1 to 2 wks, darker and thinner
    - Lochia alba: Several wks, yellowish-white color
- Adnexa
  - ◆ Bimanual palpation for any masses

A   **4- to 6-wk postpartum check**

P   **Prescribe contraception**

General rule for resumption of ovulation depends on lactation status:

- Nonlactating mothers → 4 wks
- Lactating mothers (regular, with short intervals) → 6 months

See individual Family Planning SOAP notes for more detail.

- Barrier method
  - ◆ Popular postpartum contraception
- Hormonal methods
  - ◆ Can be started within the first few wks postpartum.
    - Oral contraceptives
    - Contraceptive patch
    - Intravaginal ring
- Injectable contraceptives
  - ◆ Abnormal bleeding patterns may be confused with lochia if given too early.
- Intrauterine devices
  - ◆ Usually placed after complete uterine involution at about 8 wks.
    - Placement before involution runs higher risk of expulsion.
- Diaphragm
  - ◆ Requires involution of uterus before fitting.

Provide breastfeeding counseling

Several common complaints in the postpartum period can be alleviated with some simple interventions.

- Pain
  - ◆ Sore, cracked nipples
    - Counseling regarding infant latching/positioning
    - Air-dry nipples
    - Avoidance of creams and irritative soaps
  - ◆ Engorgement/plugged ducts
    - Frequent feedings
    - Warm compresses before and during feeding, cold compresses after
- Infection
  - ◆ Counsel pt on returning to office for assessment
  - ◆ Termination of breastfeeding not necessary

Order diabetes mellitus testing if pt had GDM

Pts who have GDM are at higher risk for overt diabetes and should be tested for glucose intolerance at their postpartum visit (see GDM p. 18).

Schedule follow-up

3 months

- For women starting new contraceptive method, schedule a 3-month follow-up to address any difficulties with usage.

Annual

- All others can follow up for their annual well woman exam.

S **Does the pt have any symptoms of anemia?**

Symptoms of anemia include:

- Fatigue   - Lethargy
- Headache   - Paresthesias
- Pica (appetite for substances of no nutritional value, e.g., dirt)

Is the pt at high risk for a nutritional deficiency?

Pregnancy may cause severe nausea/vomiting or anorexia, leading to folate deficiency.

Pts who eat diets lacking in green-leafy vegetables or animal protein may suffer from folate deficiency.

Strict vegetarians may lack Vitamin B_{12}.

What is the pt's ethnic background?

Certain ethnicities are at high risk for inherited hemoglobinopathies:

- African American: Sickle cell
- Asian/Mediterranean: Thalassemia

Is the pt taking prenatal vitamins and iron supplementation?

All pregnant pts should be encouraged to take supplemental iron and vitamins (source of folate) during pregnancy.

- Supplemental folate is most critical during early pregnancy.
  - RDA: 400 μg folate
- Supplemental iron is most critical after 20 wks.
  - RDA in uncomplicated pregnancy: 30 mg of elemental iron
  - RDA in multiple gestations or large patients: 60 mg of elemental iron

Persistent anemia despite supplementation should alert clinician to the possibility of a hereditary anemia.

O **Perform physical exam**

Physical signs of iron deficiency include:

- Glossitis   - Pallor
- Cheilitis   - Koilonychia

What are the results of the pt's Hb/Hct and mean corpuscular volume (MCV)?

Normal Hb/Hct falls during pregnancy because of a greater increase of plasma volume (50%) relative to red blood cell mass (30%).

Iron-deficiency anemia and thalassemias usually have a lowered MCV.

What are the results of the serum ferritin?

Serum ferritin reflects the amount of iron stored in the body's tissues and is the best indicator of the degree of anemia in pregnancy.

- Normal ferritin levels in pregnancy are 55–70 μg/L.
  - Low ferritin is consistent with iron deficiency.
  - Normal ferritin is seen with *early* iron deficiency, thalassemias, or chronic disease.

Peripheral smear

Morphologic features of iron-deficiency anemia (microcytosis and hypochromia) are not as commonly seen as in the nonpregnant state.

For African-American pts, what is the result of the Hb electrophoresis?

Hb S should be obtained at their first visit (if missed, obtain now).

Anemia

Anemia during pregnancy is usually defined according to the 5th percentile hemoglobin values for pregnancy (pts with values below the 5th percentile are considered anemic).
- 5th percentile values of Hb during pregnancy are:
  - First trimester   11.0 g/dL
  - Second trimester   10.5 g/dL
  - Third trimester   11.0 g/dL

Iron-deficiency anemia is the etiology in 75% of cases in pregnancy.

Inadequate folate is the second most common nutritional deficiency.

Other causes include:
- Anemia of chronic disease
- Hereditary anemias
  - Hemoglobinopathies
  - Thalassemias

 Begin anemia treatment with empiric iron therapy

Because iron deficiency is the most likely etiology of anemia in pregnancy, start with empiric iron therapy.
- Iron-deficiency anemia requires 200 mg of elemental iron/day and can be given as any of the following:
  - Ferrous gluconate 325 mg (37–39 mg elemental iron)
  - Ferrous sulfate 325 mg (60–65 mg elemental iron)
  - Ferrous fumarate 325 mg (107 mg elemental iron)

Monitor response with reticulocyte count

Normally, a response to iron therapy in the form of an increased reticulocyte count can be observed 1 wk after starting therapy.
- Response to treatment may take longer than in nonpregnant states.
  - An Hb response may be masked by physiologic progressive increases in plasma volume, which accompany normal pregnancy.
    - If present, an increase in Hb (1–2 g/dL) will be evident by 4 wks.
  - With severe megaloblastic anemia, plasma volume is relatively decreased compared to a normal pregnancy, and treatment of the anemia can be associated with increases in volume that mask rising hemoglobin.

Work up nonresponders for other types of anemia

Serum electrophoresis may reveal thalassemia.

S **Does the pt have an *obstetrical* history suspicious for antiphospholipid syndrome (APS)?**

The following obstetrical outcomes can be associated with APS:
- Recurrent pregnancy loss (three or more first trimester spontaneous abortions (SABs) with no more than one live birth or unexplained second or third trimester loss)
- Severe preeclampsia at <34 wks' gestation
- Intrauterine growth restriction (IUGR) or uteroplacental insufficiency in the second or early third trimester

Does the pt have a past *medical* history suspicious for APS?

The following medical problems can be associated with APS:
- Nontraumatic arterial or venous thromboembolism
- Stroke, transient ischemic attack, or amaurosis fugax in a reproductive-age woman
- Systemic lupus erythematosus
- Hemolytic anemia or autoimmune thrombocytopenia

O **Does the patient's skin show evidence of livedo reticularis?**

This is a skin condition associated with APS characterized by reddish-blue skin changes visible on the extremities and intensified by exposure to cold.

Do the laboratory tests show thrombocytopenia or anemia?

Although both of these disease states have multiple etiologies, consideration should always be given to the association between APS and autoimmune thrombocytopenia or hemolytic anemia.

Does the patient have a false-positive serologic test for syphilis?

Patients with a false-positive rapid plasma reagin (RPR) should have testing for antiphospholipid antibodies (see Vulvar Ulcers p. 112)

What are the interpretations of the APS serologic tests?

Two main tests are used to detect the presence of antiphospholipids:
- *Lupus anticoagulant* (LAC) is a functional assay "phenomenon" whereby coagulation is prolonged in vitro (even though thrombosis is promoted in vivo).
  - Multiple LAC assays are currently available:
    - Activated partial thromboplastin time
    - Dilute Russell viper venom time
    - Kaolin clot time
  - Results are reported as positive or negative.
- *Anticardiolipin antibody* test is an enzyme-linked immunosorbent assay test that detects antiphospholipids directed against cardiolipin.
  - Results are measured for IgM and IgG and are reported as low-positive, medium-positive, or high-positive. Low-positive results or isolated IgM are of questionable relevance and are not considered diagnostic.

A **Antiphospholipid Syndrome**
Diagnosis is made by the presence of *both* of the following:
- Any of the above clinical features
- Positive testing for antiphospholipid antibodies

P **Educate patient regarding obstetric complications (and their symptoms) associated with APS**
Pregnancies affected by APS are at high risk for:
- Placental abruption
- Preterm delivery
- Preeclampsia

Pts should be given strict precautions about the *symptoms* of these potential complications:
- Painful bleeding (abruption)
- Preterm UCs (preterm delivery)
- H/As, visual or epigastric complaints (preeclampsia)

Start anticoagulation
Treatment is based on clinical history.
- For patients with a history of fetal death or recurrent abortion:
  - Daily low-dose aspirin
  - Daily heparin in prophylactic doses (5,000–10,000 U bid)
  - PTT monitoring is not necessary.
- For patients with a history of thrombosis or stroke:
  - Daily low-dose aspirin
  - Heparin to achieve full anticoagulation (10,000 U bid to tid)
  - PTT prolongation of 1.5–2.5 baseline
  - Heparin-induced thrombocytopenia may occur with full-dose heparin.
  - Check platelet counts on day 5 and periodically for first two wks.
  - Heparin-induced osteoporosis can occur after 7 wks of use.

Serial fetal ultrasounds for growth every 4 to 6 wks starting at 18 to 20 wks' gestation
Pregnancies affected by APS are at high risk for IUGR.

AP testing beginning at 30 to 32 wks' gestation
Pregnancies affected by APS are at high risk for abnormal fetal heart rate patterns.

S **Perform a thorough review of the pt's asthma history**
This information can be helpful in making management decisions.
- What is the duration of disease?
  - New-onset wheezing should raise suspicion for other possible etiologies such as heart disease.
- How often are exacerbations?
- What are current and past medications?
- Any history of hospitalizations or intubations?

O **Check VS**
Note presence of tachypnea.
Fever can reflect an ongoing infection.

Perform PE
General
- Presence of cyanosis?
- Able to communicate in complete sentences without pausing for air?
- Able to ambulate?

Lungs
- Is there labored breathing?
- Prolonged expiration?
- Use of accessory muscles?

Review pt's peak expiratory flow rate (PEFR) values
PEFR is a quick, objective test of the pt's current respiratory function.
- It consists of having the pt exhale as strongly as possible into a plastic meter.
PEFR values also give the physician objective data to follow between clinic visits and in making management decisions during exacerbations.
- Monitoring and recording PEFR values in the clinic reinforces technique and encourages home use of this test.

A **Asthma**
Most asthmatics are diagnosed before pregnancy.
- Differential diagnosis of new-onset asthma in pregnancy is:
  - CHF   - Pulmonary edema
  - PE   - Pneumonia
  - Bronchitis   - Mechanical obstruction of airways
Asthma in pregnancy is classified as mild, moderate, or severe.
- Mild Asthma
  - Brief, episodic exacerbations with PEFR > 80% baseline
- Moderate Asthma
  - > 2 exacerbations/wk, which may last several days; occasional ER visits; and PEFR 60% to 80% baseline
- Severe Asthma
  - Continuous symptoms with limited activity, frequent exacerbations, and occasional hospitalizations

P **Counsel pt on asthma in pregnancy**
Focus of management is to *control the disease*.
- Stress to pt that medications are not harmful to fetus.

In general, there are minimal increases in perinatal morbidity and mortality and minimal changes in disease severity during pregnancy.

- One-third of pts improve, one-third worsen, and one-third do not change.

Treat chronic asthma with metered-dose inhalers

Treatment of asthma in pregnancy is based on the principle that the benefits of adequate treatment outweigh any risks of medication side effects or possible teratogenicity. Therefore, generally treat pt the same way as in the nonpregnant state.

- Mild disease is treated with inhaled β-adrenergic agonists.
  - Albuterol 2 puffs q 3 to 4 hrs PRN
- Moderate disease is treated with inhaled β-adrenergic agonists and inhaled steroids.
  - Albuterol 2 puffs q 3 to 4 hrs PRN
  - Beclomethasone 2 to 5 puffs bid to qid
- Severe disease is treated with inhaled β-adrenergic agonist, inhaled steroids, inhaled cromolyn, and oral steroids.
  - Albuterol 2 puffs q 4 hrs PRN
  - Beclomethasone 2 to 5 puffs bid to qid
  - Cromolyn sodium 2 puffs qid
  - Prednisone 40 mg PO q day for 1 wk then taper

Consider hospitalization for acute exacerbations

Monitor oxygenation

- Keep pulse ox saturation > 95%.
- Use ABG to assess carbon dioxide clearance and need for intubation.

Medicate

- Beta-agonists
  - Albuterol 2.5 mg (0.5 cc of 0.5% solution diluted with 2 to 3 cc NS)
    - May repeat q 20 to 30 minutes
- IV steroids
  - Methylprednisolone 60–80 mg IV bolus q 6 to 8 hrs
    - Minimal effects on fetus secondary to poor crossing of placenta

Consider CXR

- Obtain CXR in presence of fever, elevated WBCs, or clinical evidence of upper respiratory infection.

Consider antibiotics

Consider admission

- Threshold for admission should be lower during pregnancy.
  - Admit for PEFR < 40% after 1 hr or < 80% after 4 hrs of observation.

In labor, consider IV steroids and avoid prostaglandin F2α

Patients who have used oral steroids for $\geq$ 1 wk in the past 12 months require "stress-dose" steroids in labor.

- Hydrocortisone 100 mg IM q 6 hrs during labor

Prostaglandin F2α, used for postpartum hemorrhage, can worsen asthma and should be avoided.

S   **Has the pt been previously diagnosed with chronic hypertension (CHTN)?**
Review history, prior workup, and any complications (e.g., myocardial infarction, end-organ involvement).
With many pts, pregnancy is the first entry into the health care system and an opportunity to discover such chronic problems as hypertension.
- Previously undiagnosed CHTN mandates a full workup (see below).

Is the pt currently taking any antihypertensive medications?
Review current and past medications, doses, and length of use.
- Angiotensin-converting enzyme inhibitors are contraindicated during pregnancy because they can have teratogenic renal effects.

What is the pt's current activity level?
Activity restriction should be applied during pregnancy to avoid decreased placental perfusion.

O   **Check BP**
BP measurements should be performed serially over periods of time to establish diagnosis and confirm degree of disease.
Severe CHTN (SBP $\geq$ 180 mm Hg or DBP $\geq$ 110 mm Hg) should alert clinician to possible reversible causes (see below).

Perform PE
Check for differences between radial and femoral pulses.
- Coarctation of the aorta is a rare, but easily detectable cause of hypertension.
Check for signs of Cushing's syndrome.
- Thinning of skin, bruising, and muscle weakness/atrophy

What are the latest U/S results?
An early U/S (< 20 weeks) establishes accurate dating of the pregnancy.
- This information is useful in managing complications associated with CHTN (pregnancy-induced hypertension [PIH], preterm labor [PTL]), which arise later in pregnancy.
- Comparison of subsequent U/S to this baseline is useful in evaluating suspected intrauterine growth restriction (IUGR).

Consider evaluation of renal function
Urine analysis to detect proteinuria
Serum creatinine to evaluate renal insufficiency
- Renal insufficiency places the pt at greater risk for fetal loss and developing superimposed preeclampsia.
Doppler flow studies to detect renal artery stenosis

Consider lab studies to detect *primary* causes of CHTN
Potassium
- Low in hyperaldosteronism
24-hour urinary catecholamines
- Elevated with pheochromocytoma
Dexamethasone suppression test
- Elevated plasma cortisol suggests Cushing's syndrome

A Chronic Hypertension

Mild CHTN
- SBP ≥ 140 mm Hg or DBP ≥ 90 mm Hg before 20 wks' gestation

Severe CHTN
- SBP ≥ 180 mm Hg or DBP ≥ 110 mm Hg before 20 wks' gestation

Reversible causes of hypertension should always be considered as etiologies and include:

     - Renal disease   - Cushing's syndrome
     - Pheochromocytoma   - Primary aldosteronism
     - Coarctation of the aorta

P Monitor BP serially and determine need for therapy

BP is physiologically lowered during normal pregnancy, so patients with mild CHTN (most affected pregnancies) can sometimes discontinue medications and be followed closely.

- The primary purpose of BP surveillance and control is for maternal benefit (avoiding end-organ damage).

- Even though CHTN is associated with increased risk of preterm birth, placental abruption, superimposed preeclampsia, IUGR, and fetal death, treatment does NOT appear to reduce perinatal morbidity.

Treatment is customarily initiated for SBPs > 180 mm Hg or DBPs > 110 mm Hg.
- Methyldopa has been the most widely studied antihypertensive used during pregnancy and is recognized as safe.
  - ✦ Methyldopa 250 mg bid (max 2 g/day)
- Labetalol is also popular and safe.
  - ✦ Labetalol 100 mg bid (max 2400 mg/day)

Obtain 24-hr urine

A 24-hr urinary protein collection will reveal any underlying proteinuria.
- A baseline value (early in pregnancy) often helps evaluate for superimposed preeclampsia if signs develop later in pregnancy.

Refer to appropriate specialists

End-organ damage should be evaluated, especially with long-standing disease.
- Refer pt to cardiologist, nephrologist, and ophthalmologist to assess the respective organ systems.

Monitor for signs of superimposed preeclampsia

Superimposed preeclampsia affects 25% of pregnancies with CHTN.
- Monitor BP weekly beginning at 30 wks.

Consider AP testing

Indications for AP testing should be individualized.
- Initiate for signs of IUGR or preeclampsia.

Consider early delivery

Early delivery should be initiated for severe, uncontrolled CHTN or pts with prior bad obstetrical outcome.

S   **Is the pt at high risk for gestational diabetes mellitus (GDM) *by history*?**
A history of any of the following places the pt at high risk for GDM and warrants first trimester screening:
- A history of glucose intolerance
- A history of an adverse obstetric outcome usually associated with GDM, such as:
  - ◆ Macrosomia
  - ◆ Congenital anomalies (especially neurologic and cardiac defects)
  - ◆ Unexplained fetal demise
- A first-degree relative with diabetes

O   **Does the pt have any *objective evidence* to place her at high risk for GDM?**
Any of the following objective findings place the pt at higher risk for GDM and warrant first trimester screening:
- Hypertension
- Obesity (BMI > 30)
- Advanced maternal age (≥ 35 y/o)
- Glycosuria on the office urine dip

What is the result of the 1-hr glucose challenge test (GCT)?
Screening for GDM is done with a 1-hr GCT.
- Perform at 24 to 28 wks for pts without risk factors (see above).
- The test consists of the pt ingesting a 50-g glucose load, usually in the form of a liquid suspension.
- One hour later, the pt's venous glucose level is measured.
- The pt does NOT need to be in the fasting state to perform the test.

  - ◆ An abnormal 1-hr GCT is 140 mg/dL or higher.
    - ◆ Some clinics use a cutoff value of 130 mg/dL, which improves sensitivity of the test.

All pts with an abnormal 1-hr GCT require a 3-hr glucose tolerance test (GTT).

What is the result of the pt's 3-hr GTT?
Diagnosis of GDM is done with the 3-hr oral GTT.
- This test consists of the pt ingesting 100 g of glucose.
- Venous glucose is measured during the fasting state and at 1, 2, and 3 hrs after intake.
- Pts must be fasting and have eaten an unrestricted diet for 3 days before test.
- Pts must be sitting during the test.

Values that *exceed* the following are considered abnormal:
- Fasting   95 mg/dL
- 1 hr   180 mg/dL
- 2 hr   155 mg/dL
- 3 hr   140 mg/dL

A pt with two or more abnormal values meets the diagnosis of GDM.

Review pt's blood sugar log book
Once diagnosis is made, sugar values are usually monitored and recorded in a log book. On every visit, the log book should be reviewed and the data recorded.
- Management decisions are based on trends (see below).

A **Gestational Diabetes Mellitus (GDM)**
GDM is a form of glucose intolerance that results from the anti-insulin action of human placental lactogen, a pregnancy hormone.
GDM is divided into two subgroups, A1 and A2, which are differentiated on the pt's fasting and postprandial blood sugars and the need for insulin.
   - A1 GDM: *Therapeutic diet* controls fasting blood sugars to < 95 and the 2-hr postprandial blood sugars to < 120.
   - A2 GDM: Pt cannot maintain these target values of fasting blood sugars < 95 and 2-hr postprandial blood sugars < 120 with dietary therapy and *insulin is initiated*.

P **Start pt on dietary therapy, with total daily calories equaling 30 kcal/kg**
A nutritional counselor can be involved to individualize therapy.
Protocols for assessing blood sugar control vary from obtaining weekly fasting blood sugar values to qid home monitoring.

Monitor blood sugars
Blood sugars are either self-monitored (by pt at home) or monitored by weekly fasting blood draw (in office).
   - Self-monitored sugars are checked and recorded qid (fasting and 2 hrs after each meal).
   - Results are logged on a piece of paper to observe trends.

Start insulin for pts who have failed dietary therapy
Dietary therapy is usually considered failed when pt cannot keep fasting sugars < 95 or 2-hr postprandial sugars < 120 for 2 wks.
To start insulin, first *calculate the total daily insulin* requirement, which is based on pt weight in kg and gestational age as follows:
   - First trimester   0.7 Units/kg
   - Second trimester   0.8 Units/kg
   - Third trimester   0.9 Units/kg
Next, *divide the total daily insulin* requirement into two doses as follows:
   - Morning shot (2/3 of total daily)   2/3 NPH and 1/3 Regular insulin
   - Evening shot (1/3 of total daily)   1/2 NPH and 1/2 Regular insulin

Ultrasound
Anatomic survey at 18 to 20 wks
Consider serial ultrasounds to determine growth.

Start AP testing on A2 at 32 wks
Twice-weekly AP testing should be started on all A2 GDM pts (see Third Trimester Visit p. 6).

Scan A2 for estimated fetal weight (EFW) at 38 to 39 wks
A2 GDM pts have an increased risk of macrosomia and require a U/S for EFW at term.

Deliver A2 at 38 to 39 wks
Generally deliver A2 DM at 38 to 39 wks.

Deliver A1 at 41 wks

S **Does the patient complain of any symptoms commonly associated with hyperthyroidism?**

- Fatigue
- Palpitations
- Tremor
- Diarrhea
- Sweating
- Weight loss or no weight gain
- Visual complaints
- Anxiety

Did the patient have similar complaints *before* becoming pregnant?

Many complaints associated with hyperthyroidism can also be common to a normal pregnancy.

Ascertaining whether pt experienced these complaints before pregnancy may help distinguish etiology.

Additionally, in the first trimester, some normal pregnancies suffer from *transient hyperthyroidism*.

This phenomenon is secondary to the presence of human chorionic gonadotropin (hCG), a pregnancy hormone, which cross-reacts with the thyroid-stimulating hormone (TSH) receptor, to cause increased production of thyroid hormone.

This reaction peaks at around 10 wks with the natural plateau in hCG levels and declines thereafter.

If pt has a *history* of hyperthyroidism, what is the etiology?

95% of pregnant women with hyperthyroidism have *Graves' disease*.

This disease is characterized by TSH receptor antibodies (TSHR-Abs), auto antibodies that react with the TSH receptor to stimulate thyroid hormone production.

TSHR-Abs need to be monitored in most Graves' pts during pregnancy (see below).

O **Review vital signs**

Tachycardia and weight loss (or no weight gain) are two of the most supportive signs of hyperthyroidism in pregnancy.

Presence of fever or a widened pulse pressure should alert the physician to the possibility of thyroid storm.

Does the pt exhibit any signs of hyperthyroidism on physical exam?

- Goiter
- Hand tremor
- Lid lag
- Proximal muscle weakness
- Systolic flow murmur
- Exophthalmos
- Onycholysis

What are the results of the thyroid function tests?

Physiologic changes normal to pregnancy can alter certain thyroid function tests (Table 1).

- High levels of estrogen stimulate production of thyroid-binding globulin, which normally binds thyroid hormone.

Table I				
	TSH	Free T3 & T4	Total T4 & T3	T3 resin uptake
Pregnancy	↔	↔	↑	↓
Hyperthyroidism	↓	↑	↑	↓
Hypothyroidism	↑	↓	↓	↑

- This, in turn, raises total T3 and T4, making interpretation of these values unreliable during pregnancy.
- TSH, free T3, and free T4 (the active hormones) are unaltered.

For pts with new-onset hyperthyroidism, are TSHR-Abs present?
Presence of TSHR-Abs confirms Graves' disease.

For pts with Graves' disease being currently medically treated or those previously treated with radioiodine or surgery, what are the titers of TSHR-Abs?
Even in the face of controlled or previously treated Graves' disease, there may be high titers of TSHR-Abs in maternal serum.

High titers of TSHR-Abs can cross the placenta and react with the fetal thyroid gland to cause neonatal hyperthyroidism (rare).
- Screen for such affected pregnancies by monitoring fetal heart rate for tachycardia and documenting fetal growth (see more below).

Hyperthyroidism
The diagnosis of hyperthyroidism is made by detecting *low* TSH along with *elevated* free T3 and free T4.

Diagnosis of Graves' disease is supported by findings of a goiter and ophthalmopathy and is confirmed by detection of TSHR-Abs.
- Differential diagnosis includes:

- Toxic multinodular goiter	- Toxic adenoma
- Thyroiditis	- Hyperemesis gravidarum (see p. 28)
- Exogenous thyroid hormone	- Gestational trophoblastic disease (see p. 125)

Start antithyroid medication for newly diagnosed pts
The thioamides, methimazole and propylthiouracil (PTU), are the two currently accepted treatments for hyperthyroidism in pregnancy.

PTU is the preferred medication because of less transplacental passage.
- PTU 100 mg PO tid (titrate up to 800 mg/day)

- Rare side effect: Agranulocytosis, watch for fever and sore throat

Monitor free T4 levels
Free T4 is used to monitor response to medications during pregnancy.
- Initial free T4 normalization takes 3 to 6 wks.
- Once euthyroidism has been confirmed, check free T4 values every 2 to 3 wks.
- Dosing can often be reduced as pregnancy progresses.
- One-third of patients can discontinue medication in third trimester.

Consider AP testing
Initiate AP testing for pts with uncontrolled hyperthyroidism or high TSHR-Ab titers.
- AP testing traditionally consists of a nonstress test/amniotic fluid index (see Third Trimester Visit p. 6).
- In pts with high titers of TSHR-Abs, consider U/S to assess fetal growth and to detect fetal goiter.

S   **Does the pt have any risk factors for intrauterine growth restriction (IUGR)?**

Most cases of growth-restricted pregnancies have known risk factors, such as the following:

- Previous IUGR	- Diabetes
- CHTN	- Anemia
- APS	- Other chronic illnesses (renal, pulmonary, heart)
- Multiple gestations	- Elevated MSAFP/hCG
- Low weight gain	- Smoking or substance abuse
- Malnutrition	- Exposure to teratogens
- Primary placental disease (previa, chorioangioma)	

Does the pt have a history of exposure to infectious agents?

Although accounting for < 10% of all cases, the following infections have been associated with IUGR:

- CMV	- Rubella
- Varicella	- Toxoplasmosis

Does the pt have a history of vaginal bleeding or preterm labor?

Both of these have been associated with increased risk of IUGR.

Has the pt had a previous ultrasound?

A baseline ultrasound, preferably before 20 wks' gestation, can aid in the diagnosis of IUGR by verifying that growth was appropriate in early gestation.

- Good dating of the fetus is the single most important piece of information in the management of IUGR.

O   **What are the results of the fundal height measurement?**

Fundal height (FH) measurements are performed on *all* pregnancies as a *screening tool*.
- After 20 wks, the FH in cm should equal the estimated gestational age (EGA) in wks.
  - Consider U/S if FH < EGA.

What are the findings on the current U/S?

When IUGR is suspected, serial U/S evaluations are performed.
- Several U/S parameters can be used to identify and manage the IUGR fetus:
  - Abdominal circumference (AC) or the head circumference/AC ratio

- The AC is the most sensitive single marker for IUGR.

  - Fetal weight
    - Fetal weights, plotted on a standardized growth curve, can be followed over time to assess growth.
    - A single U/S evaluation of the fetus has limited use, but IUGR is more suspect if the estimated fetal weight is < the 5th percentile.
  - Doppler velocimetry
    - Doppler velocimetry is a U/S technique that assesses blood flow through various organs.
    - In IUGR, placental blood flow *slows* and flow to the fetal brain (secondary to physiologic redistribution) *increases*.
  - Amniotic fluid index
    - IUGR pregnancies show oligohydramnios secondary to reduced perfusion of the fetal kidneys.

A **Intrauterine Growth Restriction**

IUGR is defined as estimated fetal weight (EFW) < 10th percentile.
- Because some pregnancies with EFW < 10th percentile will represent the lower end of the spectrum of a normal population, IUGR encompasses pathologic as well as "normal" small fetuses.
    - Pathologic IUGR is suspected when an EFW < 10th percentile continues to fall off the growth curve over time.
        - Growth curves have several inherent inaccuracies (heterogeneous population of the United States, no adjustment for parity or maternal/paternal height).
    - EFW < 5th percentile is associated with greater perinatal morbidity.

IUGR is classically divided into two categories:
- Symmetric, where all fetal U/S measurements are small
    - Usually occurs early in pregnancy and is associated with chromosomal or genetic problems.
- Asymmetric, where fetal head is "spared" and the rest of body measures are small
    - Occurs later in pregnancy and is the result of uteroplacental insufficiency (not enough blood and nutrients getting to fetus).

P **Perform serial ultrasounds every 2 to 3 wks**

An interval of 2 to 3 wks allows for accurate assessment of fetal growth.
- Intervals shorter than 2 to 3 wks are prone to misinterpretation secondary to the inconsistency of fetal growth and measurement errors intrinsic to the U/S.

Initiate AP testing

Pregnancies suspected of IUGR should undergo some sort of AP testing.
- Nonstress test, contraction stress test, and biophysical profile are all acceptable (see Third Trimester Visit p. 6).

Consider Doppler velocimetry

Umbilical artery Doppler velocimetry can be used to monitor the fetus.
- Absent or reversed end-diastolic flow of the umbilical artery is associated with adverse perinatal outcome.
- Normal end-diastolic flow in a suspected IUGR fetus is reassuring.

Plan timing of delivery

Timing of delivery weighs the risk of prematurity versus the risks of prolonging a gestation in a hostile intrauterine environment.
Decision is individualized and based on:
- Gestational age
- Findings on AP testing, U/S, and Doppler velocimetry
    - Generally, deliver for EGA > 34 wks or signs of advanced fetal compromise.

Consider administering steroids to benefit fetal lung maturity

If the pregnancy is likely to be delivered at < 34 wks as a result of IUGR, consider steroids.
- Betamethasone 12 mg IM q 24 hrs × 2 doses

S **What is the father's Rh status?**
Paternal Rh status can be very important in managing pregnancies affected by Rh isoimmunization.
- If father is Rh negative and he is definitely the father, there is no risk of having an Rh-positive fetus.
- If the father is Rh positive or unknown status, an attempt to determine his genotype (heterozygous vs. homozygous for the "D" antigen) can help counsel pt on chances of having Rh-positive fetus.

What is the pt's past obstetric history?
Past pregnancies affected by Rh hemolytic disease provide prognosis for the current pregnancy.
- Good prognosis for current pregnancy with history of previously mildly affected fetus.
- Poor prognosis and high potential for recurrent severe disease with a history of hydrops fetalis.

O **What is the level of anti-D antibody?**
Anti-D antibody levels (maternal serum) reflect the degree of sensitization and the likelihood that the fetus will be affected.
Following levels serially will determine the need for amniocentesis.
- Initial titer should be taken at first prenatal visit and then every 4 wks starting at 20 wks
  - Titers that are $\leq$ 1:8 may be followed conservatively with repeat titers every 2 to 4 wks and serial ultrasound examinations to look for evidence of fetal anemia (see below).
  - Titers that are > 1:8 require serial amniocentesis.

What are the results of the U/S?
Beginning in the second trimester, serial U/S evaluations are done on the fetus to detect any signs of hydrops fetalis.
- Ultrasonographic markers of hydrops include:
  - Polyhydramnios   - Pericardial and pleural effusions
  - Hepatosplenomegaly   - Bowel edema

What are the results of the amniocentesis?
Serial amniocentesis can begin at about 24 wks in pregnancies *with titers >1:8*.
Analysis of amniocentesis to assess the degree of fetal anemia is performed by spectrophotometric density.
- Normal amniotic fluid has a density ranging from wavelengths of 525 to 375 nm.
- When bilirubin is present in the amniotic fluid (released from affected fetal RBCs), there is an increase in the wavelength to 450 nm.
- The difference between the density at 450 nm and that of normal amniotic fluid is called the ΔOD 450.
- This value is plotted on a graph called the Liley graph (see below).

A **Isoimmunization**

Isoimmunization refers to the process whereby maternal antibodies are directed toward antigen on fetal RBCs resulting in hemolysis of fetal RBCs and fetal anemia.

- **Erythroblastosis fetalis** and **hemolytic disease of the newborn** are terms to describe this phenomenon.
- **Hydrops fetalis** is a term used to describe the end product of severe disease, which is characterized by severe anemia and secondary high-output heart failure and generalized edema.

The most common type of isoimmunization is with anti-D antibody and is known as **Rh isoimmunization**.

- "D" refers to an antigen that is part of a blood system called the Rhesus or Rh blood group.
  - ◆ Other antigens in the Rh group are "C," "c," "E," and "e."

Maternal antibodies result from exposure to foreign blood antigens from:
- A previous pregnancy with a fetus that expressed blood antigens that differ from the mother's.
- A previous blood transfusion that directly exposed the mother to foreign antigens.

P **Analysis of the Liley graph**

A Liley graph plots serial ΔOD 450 measurements against gestational age.

- Plotting serial measurements follows the trend over time and is predictive of fetal anemia.

A Liley graph is divided into thirds or zones I, II, and III.

- Zone I values represent mild disease and are usually followed up with a repeat value in 3 to 4 wks.
- Zone II values represent moderate disease and may be followed with repeat testing every 1 to 4 wks depending on the trend.
- Zone III values signal impending fetal death and require intervention in the form of blood transfusion or delivery.

Plan delivery

Mild disease
- Deliver at term.

Moderate disease
- Follow trends on the Liley graph.
  - ◆ If rising, consider early delivery.
  - ◆ If falling, consider temporizing delivery (transfusing) until fetus is mature.

Severe disease
- Consider **percutaneous umbilical blood sampling** (PUBS).
  - ◆ PUBS measures fetal hemoglobin and hematocrit directly.
    - • Guides management of unclear pictures (Zone II) on the Liley graph.
    - • Also helpful for gestations that are too early to be interpreted through the Liley curve.
- Consider intrauterine transfusion.
  - ◆ Intrauterine transfusion is used to treat the severely anemic fetus.
    - • Customarily begun when fetal hematocrit (determined by PUBS) is < 25%.

S **Does the pt have any symptoms of preeclampsia (pregnancy-induced hypertension [PIH])?**

Most cases of mild preeclampsia do not have any symptoms.
- Presence of symptoms raises suspicion for severe disease (see Severe Preeclampsia p. 32).

Does the pt have any risk factors for PIH?

- Previous PIH	- CHTN	- Chronic renal disease
- DM	- African race	- Reproductive age extremes
- Nulliparity	- Multiple gestations	(< 17 or > 40 y/o)

O **What is the BP?**

BP in NORMAL pregnancy follows a predictable pattern of physiologic changes:
- First trimester   Decrease (systolic less than diastolic, increasing pulse pressure)
- Second trimester   Nadir at 24 wks
- Third trimester   Increases to term (any rise above nonpregnant values is abnormal)

Blood pressure should be measured with a correct and reproducible technique.
- Always measure with arm at the same height as heart.
- Use appropriate cuff size.
  - Larger cuffs for obese pts (cuffs fitting too tightly can cause abnormally elevated readings)

SBP $\geq$ 140 mm Hg or DBP $\geq$ 90 mm Hg taken on two occasions at least 6 hrs apart after 20 wks' gestation meets the diagnosis of mild PIH.

Does the pt have any protein in the office urine dip or U/A?

Normally, there should only be trace protein in the urine of a pregnant pt.
Greater amounts may signify proteinuria levels that are diagnostic of preeclampsia.
- The following terminology is frequently used when quantifying proteinuria in the office:
  - 1+   30 mg/dL
  - 2+   100 mg/dL
  - 3+   300 mg/dL
  - 4+   2000 mg/dL

What is the pt's CBC and expanded chemistry panel?

The following laboratory findings support a diagnosis of PIH:
- Hemoconcentration (high or high-normal hemoglobin/hematocrit)
- Elevated uric acid

The following laboratory findings are signs of severe disease (see Severe PIH p. 32):
- Low platelets
- Elevated liver enzymes

What is the result of the 24-hr urine protein and creatinine clearance?

A 24-hr urinary protein collection will quantify any proteinuria.
- A nonpregnant pt has a 24-hr excretion of 100 to 125 mg of protein.
- A pregnant pt excretes up to 150 mg of protein in 24 hrs.

Mild preeclampsia is diagnosed when proteinuria exceeds 300 mg in 24 hrs.

A **Mild Preeclampsia**
Mild preeclampsia is diagnosed by the presence of the following:
- SBP $\geq$ 140 mm Hg or DBP $\geq$ 90 mm Hg
  - After 20 wks of pregnancy on two occasions more than 6 hrs apart
- Proteinuria of $\geq$ 300 mg in 24 hrs

P **Admit**
All pts suspected of having mild preeclampsia should be admitted and observed.

Ultrasound
Perform U/S at time of admission to confirm estimated gestational age (EGA)
- Management of IUGR is based on EGA.
- U/S can be *used* as a baseline to compare with subsequent scans for fetal growth.

Monitor BPs
Pts should have BP monitored while on bed rest.
- Monitor BP hourly early in admission and then routinely if stable.
- Serial measurements help identify any progression toward severe PIH.

Monitor for symptoms of severe PIH (see Severe Preeclampsia p. 14)
Inquire daily about any PIH symptoms that could signal worsening disease.

Follow labs and 24-hr urine collections serially
Monitor lab values at least once weekly.
- Identify any trends by charting values on a flow sheet.
- Draw labs immediately for any symptoms or signs of worsening disease.

Periodic collection of 24-hr urine monitors for worsening proteinuria.

Monitor fetal well-being
Continuous fetal monitoring initially, and then daily to twice weekly surveillance (NST) for pts who remain stable while under observation.

Consider steroids
Administer antenatal steroids for gestations < 34 wks in anticipation of an early delivery.
- Steroids aid in pulmonary lung maturity.
  - Betamethasone 12 mg IM q 24 hrs × 2 doses

Plan delivery

Delivery is the only definitive treatment for PIH.

Labor induction for all term gestations.
For preterm gestations, continue bed rest until one of two outcomes is reached:
- Disease worsens
  - Progression to severe PIH mandates delivery.
- Pregnancy reaches 35 wks
  - At this time, an amniocentesis may be performed for fetal lung maturity.
    - Fetal lung maturity can be demonstrated by an amniocentesis, which detects phosphatidylglycerol or a lecithin/syphingomyelin ratio (L:S) > 2.

All pts should receive magnesium sulfate ($MgSO_4$) while *in labor* to prevent seizures.
- 4 g IV load and then continuous push at 2 g/hr
  - Toxicity can be monitored clinically by checking for decreased deep tendon reflexes and pulmonary edema.
  - Use caution with renal insufficiency ($MgSO_4$ is excreted by the kidneys).
    - Monitor IV fluid input and urine output closely.

S Obtain general history of complaint

Onset
- *Onset* of nausea and vomiting after 10 wks is unusual and requires a workup for etiologies other than pregnancy.

Duration
Frequency
Ability to "hold down" any intake

Does the pt have any associated abdominal pain, fever, or headaches?

Pain other than that associated with retching or gastric reflux from vomiting suggests an abdominal process independent of pregnancy.
Fever also suggests an alternate etiology.

- Pyelonephritis, which is common to pregnancy, can sometimes present initially as nausea and vomiting.

Headaches may suggest a central nervous system process.

Are there any specific offending agents?

Certain foul smells can cause a reflex nausea response.
Prenatal vitamins and iron preparations can also trigger nausea.

Is the nausea and vomiting affecting daily activities with family or employment?

The response to this question will give the practitioner an idea of the severity of the problem and guide treatment.
This is also a good opportunity to invite the pt's partner to become involved in the pt's care by attending the prenatal visits.

- Support at home can improve outcome.

O Does the patient have evidence of weight loss, fever, or ketonuria?

Fever, as previously stated, should not be associated with NVP.
Weight loss (or no weight gain) and ketonuria are signs of more severe disease.

Perform PE

Neck
- Check for presence of goiter.

Abdomen
- More than mild tenderness is suspicious for GI process.

Neurologic
- Check for mass lesion effect (focal neurologic deficits).

Obtain CBC, CMP, amylase, and lipase

A pt with nausea and vomiting of pregnancy (NVP) may exhibit several laboratory abnormalities that can be confused with other disease states:
- Bilirubin can be up to 4 mg/dL.
- Amylase can be up to 900 U/L.
- TSH is suppressed secondary to the high levels of hCG in pregnancy.
  - If TSH is > 2.5 μ U/mL, suspect hypothyroidism.

Confirm viable intrauterine pregnancy (IUP)

Refractory or severe NVP can be associated with gestational trophoblastic disease.
- If EGA is > 10 wks, perform Doppler tones.
- If EGA is < 10 wks, perform U/S.

Nausea and Vomiting of Pregnancy (NVP)
NVP is classified as mild, moderate, or severe.
- Classification is based on:
  - Impact on daily life
  - Weight (lack of gain or loss of) and presence of ketonuria

Mild NVP
- No effect on home life or employment

Moderate NVP
- Some interference with home life or employment

Severe NVP or hyperemesis gravidarum
- Evidence of weight loss (exceeding 5% of prepregnancy weight), ketonuria, or refractory vomiting necessitating IV hydration or hospitalization

 Mild to moderate NVP
NVP should be controlled early to avoid worsening of symptoms.
Outpatient treatment can start with conservative measures followed by various pharmalogic agents in a stepwise fashion.
- Conservative measures include:
  - Nibbling throughout day
  - Eating bland, dry diet
  - Changing positions slowly
  - Eating high-carbohydrate, low-fat meals
  - Drinking between meals
  - Getting frequent rest
- If conservative treatment fails, initiate pharmacotherapy.
  - Choice of medicine varies widely among practitioners and institutions.
  - Options for oral medications include Vitamin B_6, dopamine antagonists, and antihistamines:
    - Vitamin B_6 10–25 mg PO tid to qid
    - Metoclopromide 5–10 mg PO tid to qid
    - Hydroxyzine 25–50 mg PO tid to qid

  - Medicines dosed "qid" should be given 30 minutes before meals and at bedtime.

Severe NVP
Usually requires hospitalization
- NPO
- IV hydration until ketonuria has disappeared
- IV multivitamins
- IV pharmacotherapy options:
  - Promethazine 12.5–25 mg IV q4h
  - Metoclopromide 5–10 mg IV tid to qid
  - Ondansetron 8 mg IV bid
  - Methylprednisolone 16 mg IV tid for 3 days, taper to lowest dose over 2 wks, maximum duration 6 wks

S **What is the pt's seizure history?**
This information can be helpful in making management decisions.
- What is the duration of disease?
- How often does the pt experience seizures?
- What are current and past medications?
- Is a neurologist currently following the pt?
- When was the last adjustment of medications?

Has the pt been taking folate supplements?
Valproic acid and carbamazepine are associated with increased risk of neural tube defects (NTDs).
Folate supplementation reduces this risk.
- The recommended amount of folate for pts taking antiepileptics is 4 mg/day.
- Folate supplementation is especially important preconceptionally and during the first trimester (the time of organogenesis).
- 4 mg/day of folate is also recommended for pts with an obstetrical history of NTDs.

Is the pt sure about her last menstrual period?
Dating the pregnancy is very important in women with seizure disorder because they are at increased risk for intrauterine growth restriction (IUGR).

O **What is the pt's current drug level?**
Antiepileptic drug levels undergo complex changes during pregnancy secondary to decreases in albumin, along with increases in other plasma proteins.
- Overall, *total* drug levels tend to fall while *free* drug levels may rise.
Levels should be checked at least once at the beginning of each trimester and as frequent as each month.
- Some antiepileptics have very long half-lives ($t_{1/2}$ of phenobarbital is 100 hrs); therefore, too-frequent surveillance can lead to too much dose adjustment.
- Levels should be drawn just before next dose (trough).
  - For highly protein-bound drugs (phenytoin, carbamazepine, and phenobarbital), *free* levels should be drawn.
  - For minimally bound drugs, *total* levels can be drawn.

What is the result of the pt's triple screen? (see Second Trimester Visit p. 4)
Because of the association between antiepileptic medications and NTDs, the maternal serum alpha-fetoprotein (MSAFP) screening test should not be missed.

What are the results of the U/S survey of fetal anatomy?
Many anticonvulsants are associated with congenital malformations.
- Cardiovascular malformations, craniofacial defects, and neural tube defects should be screened for by a thorough U/S examination at around 20 wks' gestation.

Is the pt's fundal height and weight gain appropriate?
Pts affected by seizure disorder are prone to IUGR.
- If fetal growth is suspected to be suboptimal, perform serial U/S to assess.

Seizure Disorder

Seizure disorders can be classified as:
- Acquired (rare)
- Idiopathic (aka epilepsy)

Counsel pt on effects of pregnancy on epilepsy

Seizure frequency usually remains unchanged or decreases.
- Medication noncompliance and sleep deprivation can contribute to increases in seizure activity.

Counsel pt on effects of epilepsy on pregnancy

Overall, most pts have uneventful pregnancy.
However, epileptic pts have higher rates of:
- Stillbirth
- IUGR
- Preeclampsia

Continue current medication(s)

The main focus of management is to *control maternal seizures.*
Teratogenicity is of secondary concern.
- If pt begins pregnancy with a single medication that is controlling the seizures (but known to be teratogenic), it is safer to leave the seizures controlled than to switch to a supposed safer drug.

Treat with the least amount of medication possible and *avoid polypharmacy.*
If the pt has had no seizures in the previous 2 to 5 years, an attempt may be made to wean the current medication.

Monitor drug levels (see above)
Monitor pts closely for IUGR and preeclampsia

Pts with seizure disorder are at high risk for IUGR and preeclampsia.
- Document fetal growth with maternal weight gain and fundal height measurements.
  - Perform U/S if size < dates or suboptimal weight gain
- Frequent clinic visits (q week) in the third trimester to monitor BP

S **Does the pt have any symptoms of severe preeclampsia (pregnancy-induced hypertension [PIH])?**
New onset of the following findings, in the presence of elevated BP, suggests severe preeclampsia:
- Persistent, severe headaches
- Visual changes
  - Scotoma, spots
- Abdominal pain
  - Epigastric or RUQ

O **What is the BP?**
SBP $\geq$ 160 mm Hg or DBP $\geq$ 110 mm Hg taken on two occasions at least 6 hrs apart after 20 wks' gestation meets the diagnosis of severe PIH.

Does the pt have any protein in the U/A or office dip? (see Mild PIH p. 26)
Proteinuria of "3+" on office urine dip suggests that the 24-hr urine protein result will be diagnostic of severe PIH ($\geq$ 5 g/24 hrs).
- "3+" on office dip corresponds to a protein concentration of 300 mg/dL.

What is the pt's CBC and expanded chemistry panel?
Laboratory evidence of severe PIH includes:
- Renal insufficiency (elevated serum creatinine)
- HELLP syndrome
  - Hemolysis
    - Low hemoglobin and elevated lactate dehydrogenase
  - Elevated liver enzymes
    - Elevated alanine aminotransferase and aspartate aminotransferase
  - Low platelets
    - Platelets < 100,000 cell/mm^3

What is the result of the 24-hr urine protein and creatinine clearance?
A 24-hr urinary protein collection will quantify proteinuria.
- Severe preeclampsia is diagnosed when proteinuria equals or exceeds 5 g in 24 hrs.

Severe PIH

Severe preeclampsia is diagnosed by the presence of the following:

- SBP ≥ 160 mm Hg or DBP is ≥ 110 mm Hg
    - ◆ After 20 wks of pregnancy on two occasions more than 6 hrs apart
- Proteinuria of ≥ 5 g in 24 hrs
- Additional signs and symptoms (in the presence of mild preeclampsia):
    - Persistent, severe headaches
    - Visual changes
    - Epigastric pain
    - Renal insufficiency/Oliguria
    - HELLP syndrome (Hemolysis, Elevated Liver enzymes, Low Platelets)
    - IUGR
    - Oligohydramnios
    - Platelets < 100,000 cell/mm^3
    - Elevated liver enzymes

Admit

All pts suspected of having severe preeclampsia should be admitted.

Ultrasound

Perform U/S at time of admission to confirm estimated gestational age (EGA)

- Management of severe PIH is based on EGA.

Monitor BP

Pts should have BP monitored while on bed rest to confirm diagnosis of severe preeclampsia (≥ 160/110).

- Monitor every 15 minutes on arrival and then hourly if stable.

Treat blood pressure

Persistent SBP ≥ 160 mm Hg or DBP ≥ 110 mm Hg should be treated.

- Hydralazine 5–10 mg IV q 20 minutes until response (not to exceed 20–30 mg total).
- Labetalol 20 mg IV q 10 minutes up to 80 mg until response (not to exceed 220 mg total).

Consider repeating labs

For pts with abnormal results on initial labs (low platelets, elevated LFTs), repeat labs in 4 to 6 hrs to assess trend.

Plan delivery

Severe preeclampsia requires immediate delivery.

- If fetus is severely premature (< 28 wks) and pt is otherwise stable, steroids may be considered before inducing labor to aid in fetal lung maturation.
    - ◆ Betamethasone 12 mg IM q 24 hrs × 2 doses

Route of delivery depends on clinical scenario.

- Generally, pts who are nulliparous and have an unfavorable (not open or effaced) cervix should undergo a primary C/S because expedient vaginal delivery is unlikely.
- Multiparous pts with stable BPs and labs can have a trial of labor.
- MgSO$_4$ while in labor (see Mild PIH p. 26)

S **What is the pt's lupus history?**

This information can be helpful in making management decisions.

- How often does the pt experience flares?
  - ◆ Pts usually have an established pattern of either relapse-remission or chronically active disease.
- Has the pt used steroids in the past year?
  - ◆ Patients who have used oral steroids for ≥ 1 wk in the past 12 months require "stress dose" steroids in labor.
    - Hydrocortisone 100 mg IM q 6 hrs during labor

What are current and past medications?

Azathioprine and cyclosporine may be used during pregnancy.

Methotrexate and cyclophosphamide are contraindicated in pregnancy because of the risk of teratogenesis.

- These medications should be *stopped immediately*.

What is the pt's past obstetrical history?

Pts with lupus may have antiphospholipid syndrome (APS).

- APS is characterized by poor obstetric outcomes along with detection of antiphospholipid antibodies (see APS p. 12).
  - ◆ Affected pts will need specific therapy.

O **Check VS**

Watch BP and maternal weight gain closely.

- Elevated BP and/or increases in maternal weight can be the first signs of a lupus flare or superimposed preeclampsia.

What is the result of the C3 and C4 levels?

Complement levels, C3 and C4, may be followed to monitor disease state.

- In normal pregnancy, these values rise along with other acute phase reactants.
- In the event of a lupus flare, these values decline.

Follow serial measurements (rather than a single value) to detect trend.

- Check q 6 wks.

Does the pt have anti-Ro and anti-La antibodies?

These antibodies have been implicated in neonatal congenital heart block and should be tested at the initial visit.

- Affected pts should have fetal cardiac surveillance every 1 to 2 wks starting at 16 wks.

Does the pt have antiphospholipid antibodies? (see APS p. 12)

All previously untested pts should have these drawn at initial visit.

What is the pt's baseline 24-hr urine protein?

Lupus pts can suffer from nephritis and preeclampsia during pregnancy.

- Both diseases will show an increase (from baseline) in proteinuria.
  - ◆ Baseline protein excretion should be established at the beginning of pregnancy.
    - Normal 24-hr urine protein in pregnancy should not exceed 150 mg.

What are the results of the latest U/S?

Lupus pts are at increased risk for intrauterine growth restriction (IUGR) and stillbirth.

- Verify appropriate fetal growth with monthly U/S exams starting at 18 to 20 wks.

Systemic Lupus Erythematosus

Counsel pt on SLE and pregnancy

Pts may experience increase in flares during gestation.

- There is a small risk of *permanent* renal deterioration in pts with lupus nephritis.

Increased incidence of the following:

- Spontaneous abortion
- Stillbirth
- IUGR
- Pregnancy-induced hypertension
- Preterm birth
- Premature spontaneous rupture of membranes

Treat pain with analgesics

Acetaminophen is the first-line agent for analgesia.

- Tylenol 650 mg PO q6h

NSAIDs can also be used in the first and second trimester.

- NSAIDs can close the ductus arteriosus in the third trimester.

Treat flares with steroids

For mild to moderate flares, administer oral prednisone.

- Up to 30 mg/day is considered safe in pregnancy, and up to 60 mg may be required to treat severe flares.
  - Prednisone use raises the risk of gestational diabetes and preeclampsia.
  - Fetal effects are minimal, if any, because the placenta metabolizes these steroids before they reach the fetus.

Severe flares may require IV steroids or even azathioprine.

- Methylprednisolone
- Azathioprine

Monitor fetus with AP testing (see Third Trimester Visit p. 6)

Begin with weekly testing around 26 wks and increase to twice-weekly testing at 34 wks.

Consider IV steroids during labor

Patients who have used oral steroids for ≥ 1 wk in the past 12 months require "stress-dose" steroids in labor.

- Hydrocortisone 100 mg IM q6h during labor

S

Is the pt getting enough nutritional support?
Twin gestations require an additional 300 kcal/day.
Total maternal weight gain should be 40 lbs (10 lbs more than singleton pregnancy).

Does pt have any symptoms suggesting an obstetrical complication?
Multiple gestations have a higher incidence of many obstetrical complications, which
   mandates a lower threshold for working up any suspicious symptoms:
   • Pyelonephritis → Dysuria, frequency, urgency, fever, back pain
   • Preterm labor (PTL) → Preterm UCs
   • Premature spontaneous rupture of membranes → Leaking fluid from vagina
   • Pregnancy-induced hypertension (PIH) → H/A, visual changes, epigastric pain
   • Previa/abruption → Vaginal bleeding

O

Review VS
Monitor for signs of PIH:
   • Elevation of BP
   • Excessive maternal weight gain

Perform PE
Elicit two separate fetal heart tones.
   • Detection of two different heart *rates* helps distinguish gestations.
   • Inability to clearly document two viable gestations necessitates U/S.
Examine cervix if pt has symptoms of PTL.

A

Twin Gestation

P

Counsel pt on risks of multiple gestation
Counsel pt on symptoms of the many possible obstetrical complications associated
   with twins (see above).

**In the first trimester, use U/S to establish estimated gestational age
(EGA)**
Establishing an accurate EGA early in pregnancy will help in management of any
   complications that occur later in pregnancy.

In the first trimester, attempt to identify chorionicity by U/S
Identification of chorionicity is important in management of twin gestations.
   • "Chorionicity" refers to the outer membrane that surrounds a pregnancy (the
     inner is called the amnion).
   • Twins can have either dichorionic or monochorionic membranes.
   • *Zygosity* dictates which membranes occur.
       ✦ Twins can be monozygotic (which occurs when a conception of a single egg
         and a single sperm splits into two) or dizygotic (which occurs when two sperm
         fertilize two eggs).
         • Dizygotic twins always result in dichorionicity because each conception
           forms its own membranes.
         • Monozygotic twins have three possibilities, depending on how old the
           conception is when it splits (note: the amnion splits before the chorion):
             ✦ 0–3 days   Monochorionic, monoamniotic
             ✦ 4–8 days   Monochorionic, diamniotic
             ✦ 9–13 days   Dichorionic, diamniotic
             ✦ >13 days   Conjoined twins

- Monochorionic gestations are more rare but have certain serious adverse obstetric outcomes associated with them:
    - Twin-twin transfusion syndrome (when placental vascular anomalies favor blood supply to one fetus over the other)
    - Monoamniotic twins (leading to cord entanglements and stillbirths)
    - Conjoined twins

Chorionicity can be inferred by several U/S findings.

- Any of the following suggest dichorionicity:
    - Two placentas
    - Discordant fetal sexes
    - Separating membrane thickness > 4 mm (representing two amnions/two chorions)
    - "Twin peak" sign (a triangular shape that is made as the two chorions come together and fuse into the separating membrane)

At 18 to 20 wks, perform U/S anatomy scan

Multiple gestations have higher rates of fetal anomalies.

- A thorough anatomic survey should be performed.
    - Dizygotic twins have increased chromosomal abnormalities.
    - Monozygotic twins have increased structural anomalies.

Starting at 24 wks, monitor fetal growth by U/S

Perform serial U/S (q 3 to 4 wks) to assess fetal growth and amniotic fluid levels.

- Tracking fetal growth detects complications of monochorionicity and intrauterine growth restriction (IUGR) (higher incidence in twins).

Consider AP testing

Routine AP testing of twins is not recommended.

Initiate AP testing for suspicion of IUGR, fetal growth discordance, fetal anomalies, PIH, or monoamniotic gestations.

Make plans for delivery according to presentation of twins

Twin gestation presentations at time of delivery occur with the following frequencies:

- Vertex/Vertex   40%
- Nonvertex/First twin   20%
- Vertex/Nonvertex   40%

For management concerns, presentations are placed into *one of three categories*:

- Twin A vertex, Twin B vertex
- Twin A nonvertex
- Twin A vertex, Twin B nonvertex
- Management of the 1st two categories is straightforward: category 1 should attempt vaginal delivery and category 2 should have a C/S.
- Management of category 3 depends on practitioner experience and preference:
    - Twin A can be delivered vaginally followed by breech extraction of twin B.
    - Twin A can be delivered vaginally followed by external version of twin B.
    - Both twins can be delivered by C/S.

S **Does the pt have any urethritis symptoms?**
Dribbling
Mucopurulent discharge

Does the patient have any cystitis symptoms?
The classic triad of cystitis is:
- Frequency
- Urgency
- Burning
Other symptoms include:
- Dribbling
- Hesitancy
- Suprapubic pain

Has the pt had previous urinary tract infections (UTIs)?
Pts with a history of previous infection should receive longer courses of treatment.
- Previous urine cultures may be used in selecting antibiotics.

Does the patient have any symptoms more common to a pyelonephritits? (see Pyelonephritis p. 52)
The following symptoms are more suggestive of upper GU disease:
- Fever
- Chills
- Back pain (costovertebral area)

O **Review VS**
A fever is usually not seen in uncomplicated cystitis and should alert the clinician to the possibility of pyelonephritis.
- Pts with pyelonephritis can show signs of septicemia (hypotension and tachycardia).

Perform PE
Suprapubic tenderness
Back
- Costovertebral angle tenderness is associated with pyelonephritis.

What is the result of the office reagent strip testing (urine dip)?
An office urine dip can support a diagnosis of UTI by the presence of:
- WBCs: Indicating infectious process
- Nitrites: Representing enzymatic activity of coliforms
- Leukocyte esterase: Representing enzymatic activity of neutrophil granules

What are the results of the U/A and culture and sensitivity?
U/A will give presumptive diagnosis of infection by demonstrating some combination of bacteriuria, pyuria (> 5 cells/cc urine), proteinuria, nitrites, or leukocyte esterase.
- U/A with WBC casts suggests renal involvement (pyelonephritis).
Urine culture will reveal specific organism.
- Sensitivities should be used to guide antibiotic choice.

A **Urinary Tract Infection**
Acute urethritis
Acute cystitits
Asymptomatic bacteriuria
- \> 100,000 organisms/cc of urine
- There is an association between asymptomatic bacteriuria and preterm labor, intrauterine growth restriction, pregnancy-induced hypertension, and anemia.

P **Obtain urine culture**
Urine culture confirms the diagnosis and provides sensitivities for antibiotic selection.
- *E. coli* is by far the most common etiologic agent, accounting for about 90% of cases.
    - Other pathogens include *Klebsiella pneumoniae, Proteus mirabilis,* group B streptococci, and the enterococci.
A clean-catch specimen of > 10,000 colonies/cc of urine is considered positive.
- A catheterized specimen is considered positive for > 100 units/cc.

Treat empirically with antibiotics
Several antibiotics covering gram-negative rods are acceptable.
- Nitrofurantoin 100 mg PO bid × 3 days
- Cephalexin 250 mg PO qid × 3 days
- Amoxicillin-clavulanic acid 250 mg PO tid × 3 days
- Trimethoprim-sulfamethoxazole-DS PO bid × 3 days
    - Avoid sulfonamide drugs in the late third trimester for potential effects on protein binding of bilirubin.

- Ampicillin is best avoided for empiric treatment because 25% of *E. coli* stains are resistant.

- For urethritis, consider treatment for gonococcus and chlamydia.
    - Ceftriaxone 125 mg IM × 1 day
    - Azithromycin 1 g PO × 1 day

Consider a WBC count
In cases where the suspicion of pyelonephritis is raised, an elevated WBC count supports this diagnosis.
- WBCs are traditionally not elevated with uncomplicated cystitis.

Follow-up sensitivities
Drug sensitivities can be followed up to ensure that appropriate antibiotics have been given.

Perform a test of cure
All pts should have a repeat urine culture performed after treatment.
- A negative repeat urine culture assures adequate treatment (test 2 wks after treatment).
    - All subsequent clinic visits should include a screen for recurrent infection with a dip for urine nitrites and leukocyte esterase.

II

Labor and Delivery

S **Notate time of onset of contractions, status of fetal membranes, presence of vaginal bleeding, and recent fetal activity**
Status of fetal membranes is important in the management of chorioamnionitis and group B streptococcus (GBS) status (see Third Trimester Visit p. 6)

Does the pt use any medications or have any allergies?
These are important answers to establish up front in case of sudden obstetric emergency.

O **What are the pt's baseline vital signs?**
Preeclampsia is often picked up at the initial assessment of labor.
Baseline vitals can be compared to subsequent values in the face of an obstetric emergency.

What is the fetal presentation and position?
Fetal presentations other than vertex generally require cesarean delivery.
Position of fetus is important in assessing *labor dystocia* (see p. 48).

What is the pattern of uterine contractions?
Uterine contractions should be noted for frequency, duration, and quality.

What is the pt's cervical exam?
Cervical exam should note dilation, effacement, and station.
Multiparous pts are frequently noted to be slightly dilated before onset of labor.
Membranes status can be noted when dilation is adequate.
Presenting part can be confirmed.

Review pt's prenatal record
Note any problem list, obstetrical history, and Rh/Rubella/GBS status.

Review fetal heart rate tracing
Fetal heart rate tracings (FHRTs) are important to note upon presentation.
Abnormal patterns developing later in labor can be compared to earlier patterns to aid in evaluation and management.

The following standardized terminology should be used when describing the FHRT:

- Baseline
  - Approximate mean heart rate over a 10-minute period (round to nearest 5 beats/min)
  - Must be constant for at least a 2-minute period
    - Normal 110–160 BPM (tachycardia > 160 BPM, bradycardia < 110 BPM)
- Variability
  - Fluctuations in baseline with 2 or more cycles/minute
    - Absent, minimal ≤ 5 BPM, moderate 6–25 BPM, marked > 25 BPM
- Accelerations
- Decelerations
  - Early: associated with head compression
    - Nadir occurs with peak of contraction.
  - Variable: associated with cord compression
    - Rapid decline from baseline to nadir.
  - Late: associated with uteroplacental insufficiency
    - Gradual decline from baseline with return after the end of contraction.
    - Nadir occurs after peak of contraction.

A **Term Labor**
"Term" is defined as a gestation between 37 and 42 wks.
- < 37 wks is preterm
- > 42 is postterm
- > 40 is "post dates" but still considered term

Labor is defined as regular uterine contractions accompanied by cervical dilation or change.
- *Latent-phase labor* is defined as regular contractions with cervical dilation < 4 cm.
- *Active-phase labor* is defined as regular contractions with cervical dilation > 4 cm.

P **Initial evaluation**
Evaluation for labor can frequently pick up other indications for admission.
Initial evaluation for labor should include the following:
- Continuous fetal heart rate monitoring
  - Any nonreassuring FHRT mandates admission.
- Blood pressure
  - Elevated blood pressure suggests preeclampsia.
- Urine dip
  - New-onset proteinuria is suspicious for preeclampsia.
- Cervical exam
  - Obtain initial cervical exam.
    - If cervix is dilated 4 cm or more, pt is in active labor and should be admitted.

Observe for cervical change
In pts who are in the *latent phase* upon presentation (< 4 cm), observe pt for a short interval (1–2 hrs), and then check cervix for change.
- Absence of cervical change suggests absence of labor.

Admit
Admit pts who are in active labor.
- Start IV fluids.
  - Standard fluids for laboring pts is D5LR at 125 cc/hr.
- Check laboratories.
  - CBC, RPR, U/A, type & screen (if TOL, type & cross)

Assess labor pain periodically
Level of comfort during labor should be assessed periodically throughout labor.
A pain scale can be used to yield objective data.
Pharmacologic management includes:
- Narcotics
  - Butorphanol 1–2 mg IV q2h
- Regional anesthesia (epidural)

S **How heavy is the bleeding?**
Although subjective bleeding assessment by pt can be inaccurate, trying to distinguish amount between "a few spots" and "a gush of blood" can help guide the workup.

Does the pt feel any associated pain?
Presence or absence of pain is the primary distinguishing factor between placenta previa and placental abruption.
  • Placenta previa presents with *painless* third trimester bleeding.
  • Placental abruption presents with *painful* third trimester bleeding.

Has the pt had this complaint before? Any prior workup?
Some pts may have prior admissions and workup for a KNOWN placenta previa.
  • Review these records if available.

Has the pt had a prior U/S?
If the results of a prior U/S are available, referencing the report regarding the location of the placenta can help to quickly rule out placenta previa.

Does the pt have any risk factors for placenta previa?
      - Previous C/S
      - Multiparity
      - Previous placenta previa

Does the pt have any risk factors for placental abruption?

- Cocaine	- Smoking	- Prior abruption
- Trauma	- Multiple gestations	- Multiparity
- Uterine anomalies	- Premature rupture of membranes	
- Chronic hypertension/Pregnancy-induced hypertension (PIH)		

O **Review VS**
VS should be obtained and reviewed for any signs of cardiovascular instability (tachycardia and low blood pressure).
Hypertension (as a result of PIH or cocaine use) may be evident with placental abruptions.

Review fetal heart rate tracing (FHRT)
FHRT should be reviewed for any sign of fetal distress (late decelerations, bradycardia).
  • Abnormal FHRT signals decreased blood perfusion to the fetus, which can be seen with maternal hemorrhage.

  • Fetal distress in the face of maternal hemorrhage mandates immediate delivery.

Perform PE
Observe *external* genitalia (labia may be separated) for signs of active or recent bleeding.
  • Until placenta previa is ruled out, avoid digital cervical exam in order to prevent exacerbation of hemorrhage.

Perform U/S
Placenta previa can be diagnosed with good accuracy by U/S.
  • Note exact relation of placenta to internal os of cervix.
    ◆ Total previa: Cervical os is completely covered by placenta.
    ◆ Partial previa: Cervical os is partially covered by placenta.
    ◆ Marginal previa: Placenta edge lies next to (but not over) cervical os.

What is the result of the CBC?
Hemoglobin result after acute blood loss may not truly reflect degree of anemia if plasma volume has not yet been replaced.

Placental Abruption
Diagnosis of placental abruption is made clinically by painful third trimester bleeding.

Placenta Previa
Diagnosis of placental previa is made by U/S.

Differential Diagnoses
- Bloody show
- Vasa previa

Secure blood products
If suspicion for placenta previa or placental abruption is high, secure 4 units of packed RBCs by type and cross-match.

Immediate delivery for pts with active hemorrhage
For pts who are actively hemorrhaging (caused by either *diagnosed* placenta previa or *suspected* abruption), delivery must be executed immediately via C/S.

Admission for stable pts
Admit all pts who are not currently hemorrhaging but have a diagnosis of previa (made by U/S) or clinically suspected abruption.
Further management is individualized.
- Placenta previa
  - All term pts with placenta previa should be delivered.
    - Route of delivery depends on degree of previa.
      - Pts with either a total or partial previa require delivery by C/S.
      - Pts with a marginal previa may attempt vaginal delivery if pt and fetus show no signs of distress (absence of late decelerations on FHRT).
  - If preterm, pt may be admitted for observation.
    - If estimated gestational age (EGA) is < 34 wks, administer steroids for fetal lung maturity.
      - Steroids aid in fetal lung maturity in case the fetus needs to be delivered prematurely (high likelihood in the face of a diagnosed placental previa).
        - Betamethasone 12 mg IM q 24 hrs × 2 doses
      - If pt remains stable, observation may be continued until either delivery is mandated by further heavy bleeding or fetus reaches an EGA that allows it to be delivered safely.
        - Generally, once fetus reaches 35 wks EGA, an amniocentesis may be performed to demonstrate fetal lung maturity.
- Placental abruption
  - Generally requires immediate C/S
    - Vaginal delivery may be attempted in certain clinical scenarios (multiparous pt who is actively laboring, cervix is rapidly dilating, and FHRT shows no signs of distress.

S **Does the pt have any symptoms of chorioamnionitis?**
Maternal symptoms include fever/chills and uterine pain.

Does the pt have any risk factors for chorioamnionitis?
Risk factors include:

- Prolonged labor
- Preexisting infection
- Internal fetal monitoring
- Young age

- Prolonged rupture of membranes
- Multiple vaginal examinations
- Nulliparity
- Low socioeconomic status

O **Review VS**
Check for presence of fever.
Check for signs of sepsis (tachycardia, low BP, decreased urine output).

Perform PE
Comprehensive physical exam to rule out other sources of infection.
- HEENT: Evaluate for upper respiratory infection (URI) → Throat exudates, nasal congestion
- Lungs: Evaluate for pneumonia → Decreased breath sounds, rhonchi
- Abdomen: Evaluate for appendicitis/cholecystitis → Rebound, guarding, Murphy's sign
- Back: Evaluate for pyelonephritis → Costovertebral angle tenderness
- Extremities: Evaluate for deep vein thrombosis (DVT) → Swelling, color changes, Homans' sign

Pelvic
- Vagina: Malodorous discharge is suggestive of chorioamnionitis.
- Uterus: Uterine tenderness is suggestive of chorioamnionitis.

Is the WBC count elevated?
Elevated WBC count is consistent with infection.

- Labor itself may elevate WBC count slightly.

Assess fetal heart rate tracing (FHRT)
Fetal tachycardia often accompanies maternal fever.
Review FHRT for signs of compromise (see Term Labor p. 42).

Chorioamnionitis

E. coli and group B streptococcus (GBS), both colonizers of the vaginal-rectal area, are
the two most common microbes involved in chorioamnionitis.
- Other pathogens are anaerobic bacteria, making chorioamnionitis *a polymicrobial infection.*

Differential diagnosis includes:

- Pneumonia	- URI	- Appendicitis
- Pyelonephritis	- DVT	- Cholecystitis

P **Start antibiotics**

Broad-spectrum Abx are selected with focus on coverage of *E. coli* and GBS.
Gold standard regimen:
- Ampicillin 2 g IV q6h and Gentamicin 1.5 mg/kg q8h

Penicillin-allergic pts can receive alternatives:
- Clindamycin 900 mg IV q8h or Vancomycin 1 g q12h

Cooling measures

Initiate cooling measures for fevers:
- Tylenol 650 mg PO/PR q 4–6 hrs
- Cooling blanket

Consider workup for alternate source

Blood cultures, U/A, CXR
U/S for DVT

Consider amniocentesis if preterm

A suspected diagnosis of chorioamnionitis in a *preterm* fetus can be confirmed by
evaluating the following in amniotic fluid (not used with term, laboring pts):
- Glucose: Usually lowered with infection
- Interleukin-6: Elevated levels (very sensitive test)
- Leukocyte esterase: Product of WBC action signifying infection
- Gram stain and culture: Gram stain may miss some infections

For laboring pts, assess labor curve up to this point

If labor is prolonged, consider active management to decrease time until delivery and
risk of sepsis.

Watch for labor dystocia

Pts with chorioamnionitis have an increased risk of labor dystocia.
These pts also have a poor response to oxytocin.

Watch for PPH

Amnionitis places the pt at increased risk for uterine atony.

S **What is the patient's degree of fatigue?**
Prolonged labor can lead to maternal exhaustion and inability to complete a vaginal
  birth successfully.

How well is the patient's pain controlled?
Uncontrolled labor pain can result in failure to progress through a normal labor.

**If the pt is in the 2nd stage of labor, does she feel her pushing efforts
are effective?**
Epidural anesthesia may prevent optimal pushing efforts.

O **Review the patient's labor curve up to this point**
Note general appearance of labor curve.
  • See definitions of abnormalities below.

What is the pt's current cervical and pelvic exam?
Cervical exam should generally be performed every 4 hrs when the patient is in latent
  phase (< 4 cm dilation) and every 2 hrs in active phase (> 4 cm dilation).
  • It is preferable to have the same examiner for each "check" because cervical
    exams can be subjective, especially in noting station.
  • Pelvic exam should note any overdistended bladder or firm perineal body, which
    can both interfere with 2nd stage.
  • Rare anatomic findings that could be contributory to dystocia are vaginal
    septum, fibroids, or pelvic tumors.

What is fetal presentation?
Fetal presentations should be reconfirmed to be cephalic (aka vertex).
Note any of the following:
  • Caput succedaneum formation (scalp edema)
  • Moulding (changes in the relationship of skull bones at the sutures to
    accommodate pelvis)
  • Compound presentation
    ◆ Fetal extremity is found alongside major fetal presenting part (head).

What is the pattern of the fetal heart rate?
Fetal well-being should be confirmed before any interventions for dystocia are initiated
  (see Term Labor p. 42).

A **Labor Dystocia**
Labor dystocia is "difficult" or abnormal labor.
Normal labor is divided into three stages:
  • 1st stage is from onset of labor to complete cervical dilation.
    ◆ This stage is further divided into two phases:
      • Latent phase: 0–4 cm dilation
      • Active phase: 4–10 cm (complete) dilation
  • 2nd stage is from complete cervical dilation to delivery.
  • 3rd stage is from delivery of infant to delivery of placenta.
Abnormal labor patterns can occur at any stage.
  • Latent phase of labor is considered prolonged when it exceeds:
    ◆ > 20 hrs for nulliparous patients
    ◆ > 14 hrs for multiparous patients
  • Disorders of the active phase of labor can be divided into *arrest*, *protraction*, or
    combined disorders.

* Arrest disorders are defined as no cervical dilation for > 2 hrs.
* Protraction disorders are defined as:
  * Cervical dilation < 1.2 cm/hr in nulliparous patients
  * Cervical dilation < 1.5 cm/hr in multiparous patients
* Disorders of the 2nd stage of labor can be divided into arrest and protraction disorders.
  * Arrest disorders are defined as failure to descend past a given station for > 2 hrs.
  * Protracted 2nd stage is defined as:
    * Descent < 1 cm/hr in nulliparous patients
    * Descent < 2 cm/hr in multiparous patients

P Assess the power, the passenger, and the passage
The power refers to uterine contractility.
* Adequate uterine contractions may be assessed by frequency (> 3/10 minutes) or strength (Montevideo units > 200).

  * Montevideo units = Frequency of UCs per 10 min × Strength of UCs in mm Hg

The passenger refers to the fetus.
* Estimate fetal weight
* Position
  * Occiput anterior/posterior/transverse
* Attitude
  * Posture fetus assumes at term
    * Normal is curved spine, flexed head
    * Abnormal is some degree of head extension
* Asynclitism
  * When fetal sagittal suture is deflected away from midline of transverse axis of pelvis

The passage refers to the maternal pelvis.
* Use clinical pelvimetry to qualitatively assess architecture of pelvis.
  * Can sacral promontory be reached with middle finger? (diagonal conjugate)
  * Is sacrum concave, flat, anterior?
  * Are ischial spines average, prominent?
  * Is subpubic arch average, narrow, wide?

Consider interventions
Protraction disorders may be considered for the following interventions:
* Nonoperative
  * Analgesics for pain relief
  * Amniotomy
  * Augmentation of labor (Oxytocin)
* Operative vaginal delivery
  * Forceps
  * Vacuum

Arrest disorders generally require cesarean section.

S **When was the onset of contractions and how intense are they?**
True preterm labor (PTL) is likely to have a rapid onset with contractions similar in
  intensity to term labor.

Are there any other accompanying symptoms?
Additional symptoms of PTL include:
> - Backache
> - Vaginal spotting
> - Increased vaginal discharge

Does the patient have a history of PTL or preterm birth (PTB) with previous pregnancy?
History of preterm labor puts the patient at higher risk to have a repeat problem.

O **What are the results of the U/S?**
A comprehensive U/S should be performed.
- Fetus
  - Estimated gestational age/estimated fetal weight (EFW) is the most important
    piece of information when forming management plans for PTL.
  - Several findings contraindicate tocolysis:
    - Intrauterine growth restriction
    - Fatal anomalies
    - EFW > 2500 g
  - Note presentation
- Amniotic fluid index
  - Evaluate for preterm premature rupture of membranes if oligohydramnios is
    present.
- Placental location
- Uterine abnormalities
  - Uterine fibroids may contribute to PTL.
- Cervix
  - Cervical length can be assessed for shortening by transvaginal U/S.
  - A length > 3.5 cm places pt at low risk for impending delivery.
  - Note any funneling (as the internal os opens, the relationship of the cervix to
    the lower uterus changes from a "T" to a "Y" to a "U" shape).
  - Observe any changes with pt performing Valsalva.

What is the result of the fetal fibronectin (FFN)?
FFN is a protein found between the decidua and placenta.
- It is normally absent in cervical/vaginal secretions between 24 and 34 wks.
- Detection (by cervical/vaginal swab) during this time places the pt at increased
  risk for PTB.
  - Results are reported as positive or negative.
- Swab cannot be performed if pt had digital vaginal exam in previous 24 hrs.

What is the pt's cervical exam?
Cervical exam should be performed after sampling for FFN is done.
Note dilation, effacement, and station.

Is there any evidence of infection?
CBC should be assessed for possible elevated WBCs.
U/A should be assessed for possible infection.

Preterm Labor
PTL is defined as the onset of labor before 37 wks' gestation.
- PTL is not as easy to diagnose as term labor, and a diagnosis is often made retrospectively.
  - Management must proceed based on all findings, erring on the conservative side.
  - Customarily, cervical change while under observation or a cervical exam with a dilation > 2 cm or 80% effacement is considered diagnostic.

Etiologies include:

- Infection	- Uterine anomalies
- Mechanical factors	- Intrinsic premature activation of
- Uterine overdistention	labor by the fetus
	- Cervical incompetence

P **Start tocolysis**
A trial of tocolysis is begun in all gestations < 35 wks.
- This gestational age is empiric because, after 35 wks, the risk of the fetus developing respiratory distress syndrome (RDS) is minimal.

Contraindications to tocolysis include severe hypertension, hemorrhage, and cardiac disease.
Several acceptable tocolytics are available:
- Magnesium sulfate 4 g IV load and then 2 g IV qh
  - Watch for respiratory depression and blunted deep tendon reflexes.
  - Consider checking level if suspicious of toxicity.
  - Reduce dose with renal insufficiency.
- Calcium channel blockers
  - Nifedipine 10 mg SL × 3 load and then 10 mg tid
    - Avoid use with $MgSO_4$
- β-adrenergics
  - Terbutaline 0.25 mg SQ q 1–4 hrs (max 5 mg/24 hrs)
    - Avoid with hyperthyroidism and uncontrolled diabetes mellitus.
- NSAIDs
  - Indomethacin 25 mg PR load and then 25 mg PO q 4–6 hrs
    - Potential ductus arteriosus closure and oligohydramnios

Consider steroids
All gestations < 34 wks should receive steroids to enhance fetal lung development and minimize the risk of a preterm infant developing RDS.
- Two agents and regimens are available:
  - Betamethasone 12 mg IM q 24 hrs × 2 (Rec)
  - Dexamethasone 6 mg IM q 12 hrs × 4 (Alt)

Caution should be exercised with diabetic pts because steroids can increase blood sugar and increase the risk of pt developing diabetic ketoacidosis.

Culture for GBS and start antibiotics
Preterm infants are especially susceptible to early-onset group B streptococcus disease and should be cultured for this upon arrival (see Third Trimester Visit p. 6).
While awaiting culture results, antibiotics should be started:
- Penicillin G 5 million U load and then 2.5 million U q4h (Rec)
- Ampicillin 2 g IV load and then 1 g q4h (Alt)
- Clindamycin 900 mg IV q8h (Alt)

S **Does the pt have documented fevers?**

Pts with pyelonephritis usually present with fevers.
- Check for any other source of fever (see Chorioamnionitis p. 46).

Does the pt have any nausea and vomiting (N/V)?

N/V is commonly associated with pyelonephritis.
- Assess the degree of problem by asking when was the last time the pt ate.
- Moderate to severe N/V will have associated hypokalemia.

Does the pt have any urinary tract infection (UTI) symptoms?

Check for history of classic UTI triad:
- Dysuria, frequency, and urgency

Has the pt had pyelonephritis or UTI previously during this pregnancy?

Some pts will have had prior infections and been noncompliant with their suppressive therapy (see below).

Does the pt have any underlying GU pathology?

Underlying GU pathology predisposes pt to pyelonephritis.
- Inquire about history of renal stones, ureteral stents, or congenital anomalies of the kidneys.

Does the pt have any allergies?

Allergy history is important in selecting antibiotic treatment.

 Review VS

Document fever.

Check VS for evidence of septicemia (low BP, tachycardia, oliguria).

Does the pt have costovertebral angle tenderness (CVAT)?

CVAT is usually markedly evident.
- May be absent in very early infection.

Perform comprehensive PE to rule out other etiologies (see Chorioamnionitis p. 46).

Assess for contractions

UCs are common with pyelonephritis.

What are the results of the U/A, CBC, and CMP?

U/A is usually very "dirty" with the presence of bacteria, WBCs, nitrites, and leukocyte esterase.
- Note WBC level, which is commonly elevated.
- Pts with pyelonephritis frequently have emesis with resultant hypokalemia.

A **Pyelonephritis**

Pregnancy predisposes pt to pyelonephritis by two main mechanisms:
- Via progesterone
  - Progesterone's smooth muscle effect relaxes ureters and allows ascending bacteria to infect kidney.
- Via mechanical changes
  - Uterus rests on ureters at pelvic brim.
  - Right side is more affected by this (pyelonephritis occurs more often on the right side).

 Admit

All pts who are pregnant with pyelonephritis need to be admitted.

Start antibiotics
Antibiotics are selected to cover the most likely organisms.
- Most common are *E. coli*, group B streptococcus, *Klebsiella*, and *Proteus*.
- Cefazolin 1–2 g IV q8h (Rec)
- Gentamicin/Ampicillin (Alt)

Cooling measures
Pts with pyelonephritis can have very high fevers (>104° F).
- Interventions include:
  - Tylenol 650 mg PO q4h
  - Cooling blanket

IV hydration
Start IV hydration with replacement fluids to ensure adequate urine ouput.

Replace potassium
Potassium lost with emesis should be replaced with IV fluids.

Diet depending on N/V
In pts with moderate to severe N/V, consider holding PO intake until symptoms improve.

Monitor for signs or symptoms of fluid overload or adult respiratory distresss syndrome (ARDS)
Pregnancy is a high-volume state, which makes it susceptible to fluid overload when pts are receiving IV fluids and antibiotics.
Monitor fluid balance closely.
- Urine ouput should be maintained at > 30 cc/hr.
- Check lung fields periodically for evidence of fluid overload.
  - Get CXR if crackles are present.
- Limit IV fluids after giving 1st few liters.
Pregnant pts with pyelonephritis are susceptible to ARDS.
- Gram-negative bacteria release endotoxin when killed.
- Endotoxin damages respiratory endothelium.

Follow-up culture and sensitivity
Sensitivity to current antibiotics needs to be confirmed.
- 25% of *E. coli* is resistant to ampicillin.

Consider U/S of kidneys if no improvement
Pts who fail to respond within 48 to 72 hrs of treatment should be assessed for possible underlying pathology.
- Consider perinephric abscess or kidney stones blocking ureter.

Discharge after 48 hrs afebrile
Oral abx to *complete a 10-day course* of treatment
- Cephalexin 250 mg PO qid

Long-term antibiotic prophylaxis
All pts require long-term antibiotics in prophylactic doses for the remainder of pregnancy.
Verify sensitivities to nitrofurantoin (100 mg PO qd) or cephalexin (250 mg PO qd).

S **Obtain a detailed history of event**
What happened? How much fluid came out? Is this the 1st episode?
Has pt experienced any fevers/chills? How long ago did the loss of fluid occur?
- Prolonged rupture can lead to chorioamnionitis.
Is there a possibility that the leakage was not amniotic fluid?

O **Review VS**
Tachycardia and fever can signify infection.

Verify fetal well-being
Pt should be immediately placed on continuous fetal heart monitoring.

Perform sterile speculum exam
Check for pooling
- Pooling is the presence of a large collection of amniotic fluid in the vagina.
    - For gestations > 32 wks, collection and analysis of amniotic fluid to assess fetal lung maturity may be helpful in management.
        - Phosphatidylglycerol can be used.
        - The lecithin/syphingomyelin ratio can be affected by contamination.
Perform nitrizine test.
- Nitrizine paper is pH sensitive and will turn dark blue in the presence of a pH > 6.
    - Amniotic fluid pH is 7.1 to 7.3 and will turn paper dark blue.
    - Semen and blood also have an alkaline pH, which can yield a false-positive result.
Check for ferning.
- Swab posterior vaginal fornix and smear onto slide. After drying, slide can be examined under the microscope for fern-like pattern.
- Evaluate cervix for dilation.
    - Try to visualize cervix with sterile speculum to avoid digital exam and the introduction of infection.

Perform ultrasound
Amniotic fluid index (AFI)
- If SSE is equivocal, assess the AFI for oligohydramnios.
    - Oligohydramnios, < 5 cm of fluid, provides indirect evidence of rupture of membranes (ROM).
Fetus
- Confirm estimated gestational age (EGA).
- Measure fetal weight.
- Note presentation.
    - Nonvertex presentations have a higher risk of cord prolapse.

Labs
Elevated WBC count can be noted to support a diagnosis of intra-amniotic infection, but does not help in the absence of clinical evidence.
- Corticosteroids, as used in the management of preterm ROM, can elevate WBCs.

Consider indigo carmine
If the above tests cannot confirm diagnosis, indigo carmine dye can be injected into the amniotic cavity by amniocentesis.
- Pt is observed for passage of dye from vagina, which confirms diagnosis.

A **Premature Rupture of Membranes (PROM)**

Rupture of membranes at term (> 37 wks) before onset of labor

Preterm Premature Rupture of Membranes (PPROM)

Rupture of membranes before 37 wks' gestation

Differential diagnosis

- Urinary incontinence   - Semen
- Vaginal douches   - Cervicitis
- Vaginal discharge   - Bloody show

P **Manage PROM with induction**

If group B streptococcus (GBS) status is unknown, and rupture occurred > 18 hrs
   prior, start pt on antibiotics (see PTL p. 50).

Management of PPROM depends on EGA

If < 32 wks:

- Prophylactic tocolysis
  - Prolongs latency period (not useful once contractions have started)
  - Several acceptable tocolytics are available (see PTL p. 50)
- Corticosteroids
- Broad-spectrum antibiotics
  - Increase the latency period and may decrease neonatal sepsis
    - Ampicillin 2 g and erythromycin 250 mg IV q6h for 2 days followed by
      amoxicillin 250 mg and erythromycin 333 mg PO q8h for 5 days
- Continuous monitoring
- Strict bed rest
- Induction for any symptoms/signs of chorioamnionitis
- Watch for abruption (increased incidence with ROM)

If between 32 and 33 6/7 weeks:

- Expectant management
- Continuous fetal monitoring
  - If vertex and well-engaged, may consider intermittent monitoring after first
    48 hrs.
- Strict bed rest
  - High risk of cord prolapse, especially if nonvertex presentation
- No tocolysis if labor ensues
- Take a GBS culture and start antibiotics (see Preterm Labor p. 50)
- Induction for any symptoms/signs of chorioamnionitis

If 34 wks or later:

- Start induction
- Antibiotics for GBS up to 37 weeks (if status unknown)

III

Maternity Ward

S   **Has the pt experienced any heavy bleeding or cramping?**

Concern about heavy bleeding should prompt an objective assessment.

- Inquiry about when the current pad was last changed will help assess recent bleeding activity.

Cramping can be associated with involution of the uterus and is sometimes noticeable with breastfeeding as oxytocin is released.

- Pts requiring more than acetaminophen with codeine should be suspected of having pathologic etiologies of pain.

Has the pt ambulated?

Early ambulation reduces the risk of postpartum deep vein thrombosis (DVT) as well as postpartum bladder and bowel complications.

Has the pt eaten or had a bowel movement?

Gastrointestinal function should be confirmed.

Has the pt voided spontaneously?

Urinary function should be confirmed.

Does the pt have any questions about the delivery?

Discuss any questions the pt might have about the delivery, especially if any complications occurred.

O   **Review VS**

Assess cardiovascular stability.

Assess for fever.

Review I/O.

- Adequate urine output (> 30 cc/hr) should be confirmed because there is often increased capacity and decreased sensitivity in the postpartum period.
- The following factors increase the pt's risk for urinary retention:
  - ◆ Conduction anesthesia
  - ◆ Vaginal operative delivery
  - ◆ Uncontrolled pain from an episiotomy site

Perform PE

Breasts

- Examine for signs of engorgement or tenderness.

Current pad

- Assessing degree of saturation of current pad provides objective evidence of recent bleeding activity.

External genitalia

- Assess any abnormal swelling for a hematoma.
- Confirm that episiotomy is intact.

Uterus

- Palpation of the abdomen should reveal the uterine fundus.
- Confirm involution and firmness.

Monitor blood sugars in pregestational and A2 gestational diabetes mellitus pts

A **Postpartum Day I status-post normal spontaneous vaginal delivery**
Other types of vaginal deliveries:
- Postpartum Day 1 status-post vacuum-assisted vaginal delivery
- Postpartum Day 1 status-post forceps delivery

P **Dietary management**
Most pts can be maintained or started on a regular diet.
Pregestational and gestational diabetics should be maintained on an ADA diet.

Encourage frequent ambulation
Risk of the following postpartum complications can be reduced with early and frequent ambulation:
- DVT
- GI (constipation, bloating)
- GU (retention)

Consider interventions for episiotomy pain
Pts with persistent episiotomy pain can benefit from topical anesthetic sprays, warm compresses, and oral analgesics.

Follow-up CBC
Hemoglobin should reflect the predelivery hemoglobin along with the estimated blood loss.
Leukocytosis is common after normal delivery.

Confirm rubella immunity
Pts who are rubella nonimmune should be offered and receive rubella vaccine before discharge.

Confirm Rh status
Pts who are Rh negative and antibody negative should have an updated antibody screen during their delivery admission.
Pts who have remained antibody negative should have the infant checked for Rh status.
If the infant is Rh positive, the pt is eligible for anti-D immune globulin.
- Anti-D immune globulin is given as one vial of 300 μg.
- 300 μg of anti-D IgG can suppress immunity of up to 30 cc of fetal Rh-positive blood.

Consider lactation consult
Pts who appear to have trouble breastfeeding immediately postpartum will benefit from an early lactation consult.

Arrange for postpartum tubal ligation (PPTL) (if applicable)
PPTL can be performed any time from immediately following delivery to Postpartum Day 1.

S **Has the pt experienced any heavy bleeding or cramping?**
Lochia (postpartum uterine discharge) should continue to decrease in amount by
  Postpartum Day 2.
Cramping should be minimal and not require more than acetaminophen.

Does the pt have any breast complaints?
Engorgement of the breasts (swelling from blood, lymph, and milk) usually occurs
  around this time and can be uncomfortable.
  • Any excessive discomfort raises suspicion for mastitis or plugged duct.

Is the pt planning on breastfeeding?
Discussions pertaining to breastfeeding provide an opportunity for education and help
  plan follow-up care in the postpartum period
  • Maternal benefits include decreased risk of postpartum hemorrhage and delayed
    return of fertility.
  • Neonatal advantages include decreased incidence of atopic skin disorders,
    diarrhea, and infections (GI, respiratory, meningitis, otitis media).

Does the pt have any questions about discharge from the hospital?
Pts without complications are usually discharged on Postpartum Day 2.
  • This is a good time to discuss any questions the pt might have had about what to
    expect in the following weeks after delivery.

How is the pt's affect?
"Postpartum blues" (anxiety, sadness, or restlessness) can be expected in most pts at
  some time during the first 10 days postpartum.
  • Symptoms are transient and usually require only explanation and understanding.
Any pt with a prior *history* of depressed affect should be observed closely for
  postpartum depression, a serious complication that warrants medical treatment.

O **Review VS**
Confirm that pt is afebrile.
In preeclamptic pts, review blood pressure.
  • Pts with pregnancy-induced hypertension should have normal BPs for at least
    24 hrs before discharge.

Perform PE
Breasts
  • Firmness of breasts secondary to engorgement is common.
    ◆ Signs of inflammation (redness, heat) on nipple or skin are abnormal and must
      prompt evaluation for cracked nipples, mastitis, or abscess.
Abdomen
  • Confirm uterine firmness.
  • If the pt had a postpartum tubal ligation (PPTL), confirm that the wound is
    clean, dry, and intact.
Current pad
  • Confirm that the degree of saturation of current pad is decreasing.
External genitalia
  • Confirm that episiotomy remains intact.
Uterus
  • Confirm that involution and firmness remain.

A   **Postpartum Day 2 status-post normal spontaneous vaginal delivery**
Other types of vaginal deliveries:
- Vacuum-assisted vaginal delivery
- Forceps delivery

P   **Discharge pt to home**

Pelvic rest for 4 wks
Pt should be instructed to avoid sexual intercourse until perineum is comfortable and bleeding has diminished.
Tampon use should be avoided in pts with perineal repairs but are acceptable otherwise (provided they are changed frequently).

Schedule follow-up visit in clinic
A 4-wk follow-up visit is customary.
- Schedule appointment sooner if there were any complications during delivery or the postpartum period.
- A 6-wk follow-up is acceptable for uncomplicated pts who are breastfeeding. (Ovulation can return by 5 wks postpartum in pts who are not breastfeeding.)
- A 1-wk follow-up for a wound check is necessary for pts who have had a PPTL.

Instruct pt to return immediately for any signs of heavy bleeding, infection, or depression.

Prescribe iron supplementation, analgesics, and stool softeners as needed
Pts who are anemic (Hb < 10.0) should be given a prescription for iron supplementation before discharge.
Pts with a PPTL usually are given an analgesic preparation containing both acetaminophen and codeine.
Pts with postpartum constipation benefit from stool softeners.
- Docusate sodium 100 mg PO bid

Consider a home health nursing visit
Any pts at high risk for complications occurring before their postpartum clinic appointment should be monitored at home.
- Pts with a history of preeclampsia and delay in resolution of high BPs in the postpartum period
- Pts at risk for postpartum depression

Consider a lactation consult before discharge
Any pts experiencing breastfeeding problems will be more successful when they receive counseling before returning home.

Consider contraception
Customarily, contraception can be offered at the postpartum visit in 4 to 6 wks.
Consider offering contraception before discharge for:
- Potential noncompliant pts
- Potential fallouts
- Pts who should not get pregnant again

See individual Family Planning sections (pp. 80–90) for detail.

S **Is the pt having any symptoms other than dyspnea?**
Pts with pulmonary embolus can also experience pleuritic chest pain and apprehension.

Does the pt have a history of cardiac, valvular, or vascular disease?
Underlying cardiac disease can predispose pt to pulmonary edema.
- The postpartum period may be the first presentation of such disease.
- Pts with coronary artery disease are at increased risk for myocardial infarction (MI).

Does the pt have any risk factors for deep vein thrombosis (DVT)/pulmonary embolus?
Prior DVT/pulmonary embolus
Hypercoagulable state (familial or acquired thrombophilia)
Antiphospholipid syndrome (see APS p. 12)

O **Review delivery history**
Check for complications of delivery, which may predispose pt to some of the etiologies of dyspnea.
- Pts with pregnancy-induced hypertension (PIH) are at increased risk for pulmonary edema.
  - These pts are usually on $MgSO_4$ in the postpartum period.
    - The hypo-oncotic pressures associated with PIH and the increased fluids associated with $MgSO_4$ use place the pt at increased risk for pulmonary edema.
    - $MgSO_4$ can also directly suppress the respiratory rate.
- Pts with intrapartum infection are at risk for sepsis.
- Pts who received general (endotracheal) anesthesia are at increased risk for aspiration.

Review VS
Temperature
- Low-grade fever may be associated with pulmonary embolus
Check for tachypnea and cardiovascular stability.
Check I/O
- A positive fluid balance suggests fluid overload.

Perform PE
Heart
- Atrial fibrillation can lead to clot formation and pulmonary embolus.
Lungs
- Check for signs of pulmonary edema or decreased breath sounds associated with pulmonary embolus or infiltrate.
Extremities
- Check for signs in the lower extremities that could signal DVT:
  - Swelling
  - Tenderness
  - Homans' sign (calf pain upon dorsiflexion of the ankle)

Obtain stat pulse ox
Pulse oximetry can be used to rapidly assess blood oxygenation.
- Saturation values < 90% imply inadequate oxygenation.

A **Dyspnea**
Differential diagnosis:
- Pulmonary embolus   - Pulmonary edema
- Aspiration   - Adult respiratory distress syndrome (ARDS)
- Pneumonia   - Sepsis
- MI   - Pneumothorax

P **Obtain ABG**
PE findings include decreased O_2 and CO_2 and respiratory alkalosis.
- pO_2 value > 90 mm Hg essentially rules out pulmonary embolus.

Obtain CXR
Check for infiltrate or edema.
- Usually normal with pulmonary embolus but may have radiolucent area.

Obtain ECG
Check for ischemia or MI.
- PE findings inconsistent but can have nonspecific T-wave inversions or triad of $S^1Q^3T^3$.

Obtain CBC
Elevated WBCs are consistent with infection.

Consider D-dimer level
D-dimer level < 0.25 mg/L is very sensitive for ruling out DVT.

Consider MgSO$_4$ level
If pt is on $MgSO_4$, consider checking level for toxicity.
- $MgSO_4$ toxicity (> 15 mg/dL) can lead to respiratory depression.

Consider imaging workup for DVT or pulmonary embolus
U/S
- U/S can be used to assess DVT with a sensitivity > 90%.
Ventilation-perfusion (V/Q) scan
- A V/Q scan is used to diagnose pulmonary embolus.
- Works by detecting a difference between air distribution and blood distribution within the lungs.
Spiral CT scan
- Detects pulmonary embolus with a high degree of sensitivity.

Consider empiric treatment of pulmonary embolus
Baseline PT/PTT
Load with 7500 U heparin (70–80 U/kg) followed by 1500 U/hr (20 U/kg/hr)
- Follow PTT values every 4 hrs and titrate to 1.5 to 2.5 times control (60–80 sec)

Treat underlying etiology
Diuresis for evidence of fluid overload
Antibiotics for evidence of pneumonia

Consultation
Early consultation for management of pulmonary embolus, MI, ARDS, or pneumothorax

S **Does pt have any symptoms that may localize the source of infection?**

HEENT/Lung complaints
- Upper respiratory infection (URI), pneumonia

Breast complaints
- Abscess, mastitis

Wound pain
- Infection

Extremities
- Deep vein thrombosis (DVT)

GU complaints
- Urinary tract infection, pyelonephritis

Does the pt have any risk factors for postpartum endometritis?

Risk factors include:

- Cesarean section	- Prolonged labor
- Prolonged rupture of membranes	- Preexisting infection
- Low socioeconomic status	- Multiple vaginal examinations

O **Check VS**

Mild fever is common in the 1st 24 hours postop and of no clinical significance.
Cardiovascular stability should be confirmed by BP and heart rate.
Document all I/O.
- Urine output should be > 30 cc/hr.

Perform PE

Comprehensive PE to rule out other sources of infection
- HEENT
  - ◆ Evaluate for URI → Throat exudates, nasal congestion
- Lungs
  - ◆ Evaluate for pneumonia → Decreased breath sounds, rhonchi
- Abdomen
  - ◆ Evaluate for appendicitis/cholecystitis → Rebound, guarding, Murphy's sign
  - ◆ Evaluate for wound infection (for C/S) → Skin color changes, wound discharge
- Back
  - ◆ Evaluate for pyelonephritis → Costovertebral angle tenderness
- Extremities
  - ◆ Evaluate for DVT → Swelling, color changes, Homans' sign

Pelvic
- Vagina
  - ◆ Malodorous discharge is consistent with endomyometritis.
- Uterus
  - ◆ Check for presence of uterine tenderness, which is suggestive of endomyometritis.
    - Very subjective finding if pt had C/S (secondary to incision tenderness).

What is the result of the CBC?

Hemoglobin should reflect intraoperative estimated blood loss.
Elevated WBCs can be a result of surgery.

Endomyometritis
Polymicrobial infection with same pathogens as chorioamnionitis (see Chorioamnionitis p. 46)
- Anaeorbic bacteria are especially predominant after C/S.

Differential diagnosis
- Enterococcal infection
- Septic pelvic thrombophlebitis
- Septic shock

Start antibiotics
Broad-spectrum antibiotics are selected, including coverage of anaerobic bacteria.
Gold standard regimen:
- Gentamicin 1.5 mg/kg IV q8h and Clindamycin 900 mg IV q8h

Cooling measures
Initiate cooling measures for fevers:
- Tylenol 650 mg PO/PR q 4 to 6 hrs
- Cooling blanket

Consider workup for other sources
CXR
Blood cultures
U/S for DVT

Consider monitoring gentamicin levels
Peak and trough levels should be evaluated for the following:
- Bacteremic pts
- > 5 days of treatment
- Obese pts
- Pts with renal insufficiency

Evaluate response to treatment
Response to treatment is evaluated by defervescence.
- Response should be evident within 48 to 72 hrs.

Consider enterococcal coverage
Enterococcus is not sensitive to the gentamicin/clindamycin regimen and can occasionally be a contributory pathogen to endomyometritis.
- For pts who do not defervesce in 48 to 72 hrs, add ampicillin for enterococcal coverage.
  - Ampicillin 2 g IV q6h

Consider septic vein thrombophlebitis
If pts continue to spike fevers, consider septic vein thrombophlebitis.
- Diagnosis is usually one of exclusion, and therapy consists of empiric heparin.
  - Load with 7500 U heparin (70–80 U/kg) followed by 1500 U/hr (20 U/kg/hr).
  - Follow PTT values every 4 hrs and titrate to 1.5 to 2.5 times control (60–80 sec).
  - Continue IV heparin until defervescence.
- CT scan may provide imaging evidence of thrombus.

S   **Is the pt responsive?**
An initial observation of the pt's state gives you an idea of cardiovascular status.

Does the pt feel dizzy?
Dizziness is another subjective indicator of severity of blood loss.

Obtain history from Nursing
Nursing will be able to review the *immediate* bleeding history, pad counts, and timing
   to give you an idea of the degree of bleeding.

O   **Review delivery history**
Look for a history of lacerations or difficult placental delivery that might focus exam
   regarding etiology
The following are risk factors for postpartum hemorrhage (PPH):
   - Oxytocin use   - Tocolytic use
   - Macrosomia   - Chorioamnionitis
   - High parity   - Rapid or prolonged labor
   - Distention of uterine cavity (multiples, polyhydramnios)

Review VS
Stat VS should be reviewed for cardiovascular stability.
Urine output is the primary indicator of fluid volume status.
   • Oliguria is urine output < 30 cc/hr.

Perform PE
Adequate inspection and palpation is key to finding the etiology of hemorrhage.
   • If bedside exposure is not adequate, consider transferring pt from Maternity to a
     Labor and Delivery Room.
This also allows for the pt to be ready in case a D&C or surgical exploration is required.
   • Use a flashlight or good lighting source for inspection.
External genitalia and vagina
   • Note any lacerations.
Bimanual exam
   • Evacuate all blood clots.
     ◆ Blood clots can cause a blockage at the cervix and prevent the uterus from
       involuting.
   • Note firmness of uterus.
     ◆ A large, boggy uterus is consistent with uterine atony.

What are the results of the pt's CBC?
Noting the Hb/Hct result (from before delivery) will give you an idea of the pt's reserves.
Consider PT/PTT.

Consider U/S
If PE does not yield etiology, consider a U/S to search for fragments of retained placenta.
   • Retained products are seen ultrasonographically as echogenic foci along the
     endometrial lining (stripe).

A **Postpartum Hemorrhage**
Defined as a 10% change in Hct from admission to postpartum period or need for transfusion.
- Average estimated blood loss (EBL) for vaginal delivery is 500 mL and for C/S 1000 mL.
    - Subjective assessment of EBL is notoriously inaccurate.

The differential diagnosis for PPH in the immediate postpartum setting includes:

- Uterine atony	- Uterine inversion
- Genital laceration	- Uterine rupture
- Retained placental products	- Placenta accreta

P **Secure venous access**
Stat fluid bolus for hypovolemia

Secure blood products
Type and screen if not already done
- Cross-match packed RBCs if anticipating a transfusion.
- Transfusion criteria based on individual picture:
    - Considered for *symptomatic pts* or $Hb < 8 \ g/dL$

Treat underlying etiology
Atony
- Uterine massage and evacuation of any blood clots
- Pharmacologic treatments:
    - Oxytocin
        - 20–30 U in 1 L of IV fluids with continuous infusion
    - Prostaglandins
        - E^1 analogue 400–100 μg PR
        - E^2 dinoprostone 20 mg PR q2h (may cause hypotension)
        - F2α 0.25 mg IM or IMM q 15 minutes (contraindicated with asthmatics)
    - Methylergonovine 0.2 mg IM q2h (may cause or worsen hypertension)
Genital laceration
- Surgically repaired
Retained products
- Requires D&C (useful to have ultrasound available for guidance)
Uterine inversion
- IMMEDIATE manual replacement (may be aided by halothane for uterine relaxation)

Consider surgical exploration (laparotomy)
For unclear etiology or persistent bleeding from the uterus (suspected uterine rupture or accreta), consider laparotomy.
- Intraoperative interventions to stop hemorrhage include ligation of uterine or ovarian arteries, repair of ruptured uterus, or hysterectomy.

Consider selective artery embolization
Performed in angiography suite by interventional radiologist.
Works by catheterization of femoral artery followed by identification of bleeding artery (by fluoroscopy) and embolization.

IV

Gynecology Clinic

S When was the pt's last menstrual period, and what is her recent menstrual history?

Review menstrual history for complaints that require a workup:

- Abnormal uterine bleeding, oligomenorrhea, and amenorrhea
- Noting day in current cycle will help interpret findings on PE.

Review PMH, PSH, medications, allergies, and social history

Notate any possible drug–contraceptive interactions.

Previous gynecologic surgeries should be noted in relation to any current complaints and PE.

Review family history

Special attention should be paid to gynecologic or breast cancers.

O Perform PE

Breasts

- The clinical breast examination allows for early detection of breast cancer and other breast diseases (see Breast Mass p. 74).
- Optimally performed in 1st half of menstrual cycle

Pelvis

- Vulva
  - ✦ Inspect
  - ✦ Palpate
    - Skene's glands empty into the urethra at the meatus, which can be found anterior to opening of vagina.
    - Bartholin's glands can be palpated just inside vaginal opening on the posterior lateral portion (5 o'clock and 7 o'clock).

Insert speculum to expose vagina and cervix.

- Vagina
  - ✦ Multiple rugae or folds are visible.
  - ✦ Check for presence of discharge (see Vulvovaginitis p. 114).
- Cervix
  - ✦ External os (opening to endometrial cavity) is visible on inspection.
  - ✦ May visualize ectropion and normal amount of cervical mucus.
  - ✦ Small, white "pimples" are nabothian cysts.
  - ✦ Nulliparous cervix is smaller, multiparous larger.
  - ✦ Inspect for gross lesions or any abnormal discharge .
  - ✦ Perform Pap smear.
    - Rotate spatula twice at the external os to sample the transformation zone.
    - Rotate cytobrush once inside the os to sample the endocervix.
  - ✦ Offer STD screening.
    - For pts desiring STD screening, *N. gonorrhoeae* and *Chlamydia* cultures may be run by polymerase chain reaction off the Pap sampling.

Remove speculum and perform bimanual examination.

- Uterus
  - ✦ Palpated on bimanual examination, check for mobility, size, tenderness, contour, and masses.
  - ✦ Nulliparous women have smaller uteri than multiparous women.

- Adnexa
  - ◆ Palpated on bimanual examination, check for size, consistency, and presence of any masses.
  - ◆ Note cycle day in the presence of ovarian enlargement.
    - • Functional cysts can enlarge up to 3.5 cm.
- Rectum
  - ◆ Begin digital rectal exam at age 35.
  - ◆ Check for uterosacral ligament nodularity, which may indicate endometriosis.

Review past Paps and mammograms
Annual exam provides a good time to pick up any ongoing problems.

A
P Well Woman Exam

Annual tests
All women should have an annual Pap smear (consider longer interval if 3 normal Paps in a row).

Women > 40 should have a mammogram every 1 to 2 years.

Women > 50 should have a mammogram every year.

Contraceptive counseling
Annual exam provides opportunity to reinforce continued use in current contraception users.
- Pts not currently on contraception (or abstinent) should be counseled and offered some form of birth control.

STD counseling
Provide information on protection, partner selection, and sexual practices.

Educate pt about specific diseases, risk factors, and screening tests.

Fertility counseling
Annual examination is a good opportunity to review future childbearing plans.

Fertility declines rapidly at age 35 to 37, and efforts should be made to promote childbearing accordingly.

Women planning to conceive after age 35 need to be counseled about their increased risk of trisomies.

Dietary counseling
All women of reproduction age should be taking:
- Folate 0.4 mg daily
- Calcium 1000 mg total intake daily

Gynecologic cancer counseling
Provide information on all gynecologic cancers with emphasis on risk factors and prevention.
- Uterine cancer is the most common type of gynecologic malignancy.
  - ◆ Risk factors: Hypertension, obesity, estrogen excess
- Cervical cancer
  - ◆ Risk factors: Multiple sexual partners, early coitarche, human papilloma virus exposure, low socioeconomic status
- Ovarian cancer
  - ◆ Risk factors: Family history, nulliparity, environmental, breast or GI cancers

S **Obtain a detailed menstrual history**
Normal cycle
- Length
  - Normal cycle length is 21 to 35 days.
- Menstruation characteristics
  - Normal menstruation lasts 4 to 7 days and has an average flow of 30 cc.

Features of complaint
- Cycle changes, flow changes, intermenstrual bleeding
- Duration of problem
- Dysmenorrhea symptoms confirm presence of ovulation.

Is the pt currently using any contraception or medicines?
Contraceptive hormones, IUDs, numerous medications, and herbs can cause abnormal uterine bleeding (AUB).

Does the pt smoke?
Smoking can be an independent etiology of AUB.

Does the pt have any risk factors for endometrial cancer?
AUB is the most common presentation of uterine cancer.
The following are risk factors for uterine cancer:

- Hypertension	- Obesity
- Nulligravidas	- Long history of anovulation
- Diabetes	- Tamoxifen use

Does the pt have a history of easy bleeding or bruising?
Consider a coagulopathy as the etiology.

Does the pt have any history that precludes estrogen therapy?
Estrogen therapy plays an important role in the medical treatment of AUB.
- Smokers > 35 y/o or pts with a history of deep vein thrombosis should not use estrogen therapy.

O **Perform PE**
General
- Note obesity (BMI > 30).
Neck
- Check thyroid for presence of goiter.
Skin
- Examine for bruising, hirsutism, or acanthosis nigricans.
Abdomen
- Check for hepatosplenomegaly, which can suggest systemic disease as underlying cause.
Pelvic
- Inspect and palpate for evident pathology and possible foreign bodies.

Check labs

- β-hCG (rule out pregnancy)	- CBC (check for anemia)
- TSH	- Prolactin
- PT/PTT and Von Willebrand's disease (if coagulopathy is suggested)	
- Pap, gonococcus, and chlamydia testing (if not current)	

Consider transvaginal U/S
U/S may detect intracavitary lesion such as polyp or fibroid.

Consider endometrial biopsy (EMB)
Rule out cancer with EMB in *any pt > 35 y/o* or with risk factors.

A   Abnormal Uterine Bleeding
This is the general diagnosis given to these pts while a workup attempts to find a definitive etiology.

Possible etiologies include:

- Uterine cancer	- Uterine hyperplasia
- Polyps	- Fibroids
- Adenomyosis	- Systemic disease
- Coagulopathies	- Endocrinopathies (thyroid, prolactin,
- Infection	polycystic ovary syndrome)
	- Trauma

Many times, a definite etiology is not found, and a diagnosis of exclusion is made.
- If no apparent etiology can be found and pt has evidence of ovulation, the diagnosis can further be specified as:
  - Ovulatory AUB
- If no apparent etiology can be found and pt does not have evidence of ovulation, the diagnosis can further be specified as:
  - Anovulatory AUB, also known as dysfunctional uterine bleeding (DUB)

P   Identify and treat any underlying (organic) disease
Treat any etiology identified during above workup.
- If no organic etiology can be found, treat according to the diagnosis of exclusion.

Treat ovulatory AUB with hormones, NSAIDs, antifibrinolytic agents, or progesterone IUD
Oral contraceptives
- Numerous formulations available

NSAIDs
- Motrin 400 mg PO tid for 1st 3 to 4 days of period

Antifibrinolytic agents
- Tranexamic acid 1 g PO qid for 1st 3 to 4 days of period

Progesterone (levonorgestrel) IUD

Treat DUB with hormones
Oral contraceptives

Progestins
- Medroxyprogesterone acetate 10 mg PO for 10 days each month

Consider surgery
AUB refractory to medical treatment may require surgical therapy.
- Options include:
  - Hysterectomy
  - Ablation: The use of heat or electrical energy to "burn" endometrial lining.

S **Does the pt feel a lump?**
Pts frequently present with having "felt a lump" on breast self-examination.
  - Masses appreciated by patient and not clinician still warrant complete workup.

How long has the mass been present?
New masses are more suspicious for malignancy.
Consider fibroadenoma in an established mass.
  - Fibroadenoma is a benign, slow-growing tumor common in the reproductive years (onset usually before 20 y/o).

Has the mass increased in size?
Any rapidly growing mass should be excised, even if previous biopsy has documented it as benign.

Does pt have any symptoms associated with her menstrual cycle?
Consider fibrocystic breast disease in pts who complain of multiple, bilateral lumps that increase in size and become tender or "burn" before menstruation.

Is pt experiencing any breast discharge?
Unilateral bloody or serous nipple discharge may indicate malignancy.

Is pt having screening mammograms?
Mammograms are recommended every 1 to 2 yrs (begin screening at age 40 or 10 yrs before pt reaches the age a first-degree relative was diagnosed with cancer).

Does the pt have any risk factors for breast cancer?
Risk factors for breast cancer should be reviewed; however, all palpable masses must be worked up regardless of risk factors.
  - History of breast cancer
  - History of ductal carcinoma in situ
  - First-degree relatives with breast cancer
  - History of atypical hyperplasia

O **Perform breast exam**
Best timing is shortly after menstruation (document where pt is in menstrual cycle).
General
  - Sitting exam
    - Inspection: Note any area of skin thickening or nipple retraction.
    - Palpation: Assess axillae for lymph node enlargement.
  - Supine exam
    - Arms lifted above head
    - Palpate lightly, medium, and deeply to assess tissue at various depths.
    - Use the pads of three fingers with circular, coin-sized movement.
    - Examine a large area (from the sternum to the midaxillary line and from the clavicle to the bra line) in vertical, overlapping rows.
    - Squeeze areola to extract any nipple discharge.
Mass
  - Size
  - Consistency → Fibroadenomas are rubbery.
  - Mobility → Fixed masses are suspicious for malignancy.
  - Contour → Smooth (likely benign) vs. irregular (suspicious)
  - Skin changes → Peau d'orange (interstitial fibrosis secondary to edema)

A **Palpable Breast Mass**
Differential diagnosis includes fibroadenoma, simple cyst, fibrocystic changes, benign lesions with or without atypia, cancer, fat necrosis, and metastasis to breast.

P **Perform fine-needle aspiration (FNA) or ultrasonography**
If mass is readily palpable by clinician, the first step is differentiation between a solid (potentially malignant) and cystic (probably benign) mass.
Both FNA and U/S help qualify a palpable breast mass as cystic or solid.
- FNA uses a 21- to 24-gauge needle to aspirate tissue or fluid from a palpable mass.
  - If clear or dark fluid returns, the mass is a simple cyst.
  - If tissue or sanguineous fluid (bright blood) is obtained, specimen is submitted to pathologist for cytologic examination for malignancy.
  - Lack of any aspirate suggests a solid mass and mandates further workup.
- Ultrasonography directly characterizes size, border, and echogenicity (solid vs. cystic) of mass.
- Once detected on U/S, simple cysts may be either followed up routinely or aspirated to alleviate pt symptoms or anxiety.

Consider diagnostic mammogram
If FNA or U/S is inconclusive or *clinician* cannot palpate a mass that is apparent to *patient*, perform a diagnostic mammogram (in women < 30 y/o, U/S is preferred over mammography because cysts are expected and radiation is avoided).
A diagnostic mammogram differs from a screening mammogram in that the former requires the presence of a radiologist for immediate review and planning of further workup.
The following classification system is used in reporting mammogram results:
- Bi-Rads 1: no abnormality detected, routine follow-up
- Bi-Rads 2: benign findings, resume screening mammography
- Bi-Rads 3: most likely benign, but follow-up imaging recommended in ≤ 6 months
- Bi-Rads 4: suspicious appearance, biopsy recommended (see below)
- Bi-Rads 5: almost certainly a malignancy, biopsy/excision required (see below)
- Bi-Rads 0: used by radiologists to define an examination as inconclusive and further studies needed or old films necessary for comparison

Consider core-needle biopsy
Core-needle biopsy is performed under U/S guidance or using a stereotactic device (digital x-ray and computer-aided positioning of a biopsy gun loaded with a 14- to 18-gauge needle).

Consider open biopsy
Used for further workup of positive mammogram findings when core-needle biopsy is not available or when a breast abnormality is thought to exist, but mammogram and U/S do not detect lesion.
- MALIGNANCY IS NOT EXCLUDED with negative imaging studies.
- Up to 15% of mammograms are falsely negative, and open biopsy is needed for tissue diagnosis in the presence of suspected pathology.

S **Obtain a detailed chronologic history of the pain**
- Where exactly is the pain?
- What is the timing of the pain?
- Associated life events?
- Are there any other sites of pain, such as the back or H/A?
- Any previous medical evaluations?
- Any interventions?
- Any GI or GU complaints?

Obtain a detailed menstrual history
What is the cycle length and regularity?
Any cyclic pain?
- Pain during menses suggests endometriosis.
- Pain midcycle suggests ovulatory pain.

Is there any abnormal uterine bleeding?

Does the pt have a history of pelvic or abdominal infections or procedures?
Pelvic adhesions could be a possible etiology.

Is the pt currently suffering from any emotional or psychological distress?
Educating pts on psychological contributions to pain makes them more willing to discuss this issue.

What is the pt's social history?
- What are the pt's work and leisure habits like?
- Any major stresses as child, teenager, or adult?
- Is there current family support?
- Is the pt married? with children?
- How is the family functioning?
- Any history of sexual abuse?

Obtain a sexual history
Does the patient have a history of dyspareunia?

O **Perform generalized PE**
Assess HEENT for any neurologic source of pain.
Assess thyroid for contributory lethargy or anxiety.
Assess CVAT to rule out pyelonephritis.

Have pt identify source of pain
Have pt point to spot with one finger.
- Tender spots outside of the pelvis need to be evaluated.
  - Multiple focal tender points on trunk and extremities can suggest fibromyalgia.

Perform abdominal exam
Start with palpation of upper quadrants, looking for any hepatosplenomegaly.
Tenderness elicited from the abdominal wall can be differentiated from visceral pain by asking the pt to contract abdominal wall muscles.
- This will increase pain originating from the abdominal wall.

Examine any previous surgical scars for possible nerve entrapment.

Perform pelvic examination
Begin with external genitalia, inspecting vulva, labia, clitoral and perianal areas.
- A cotton-tipped applicator can be useful in testing focal points of tenderness.

Pts experiencing vaginismus during speculum may be relieved after contracting and relaxing perineal muscles.
Rectal exam may suggest proctitis, colitis, or endometriosis.

Obtain appropriate lab studies

WBC should be checked for possibility of infection, especially if pain has been worsening recently.

N. gonorrhoea and *Chlamydia* cultures should be obtained to rule out pelvic inflammatory disease.

U/A can rule out GU involvement.

Consider erythrocyte sedimentation rate as a marker when following pts over a period of time.

Consider using standardized psychological testing

Minnesota Multiphasic Personality Inventory

Beck Depression Inventory

A Chronic Pelvic Pain

Chronic pelvic pain (CPP) is defined as pain causing a functional disability and

- \> 3 months in duration and unrelated to menses **or**
- \> 6 months in duration and related to menses

Remember, this is a symptom, not a disease.

Endometriosis is the leading gynecologic diagnosis.

- Other etiologies include:
  - Severe dysmenorrhea   - Irritable bowel syndrome
  - Fibromyalgia   - Interstitial cystitis
  - Hernia   - Arthritis
  - Urethral syndrome   - Depression/Somatization

P Rule out nongynecologic sources of CPP

Efforts are first made to rule out nongynecologic causes of CPP.

- If no nongynecologic source is found, treatment is usually begun empirically for endometriosis.

Begin empiric treatment for endometriosis

Suspected endometriosis is initially managed with empiric medical treatment.

- Oral contraceptives
  - ◆ 3-month trial (response to them is usually mediocre)
- NSAIDs
  - ◆ Ibuprofen up to 800 mg PO q6h
- Gonadotropin-releasing hormone agonist
  - ◆ Depot leuprolide acetate 3.75 mg IM q month up to 6 months
    - • This medication works by shutting down the hypothalamic-pituitary-ovarian axis in order to decrease serum estrogen, the source of endometrial implant stimulation.
    - • Sometimes given with low-dose estrogen replacement to counter the hypoestrogenic side effects of vasomotor symptoms and bone loss.

Consider surgical intervention

Consider surgery to aid in the diagnosis of CPP.

- Surgery can also be used to treat documented endometriosis (usually resection of implants).

Consider a multidisciplinary team approach for optimal outcome

Team might include psychological and nutritional experts.

S   What is the pt's menstrual history?

Degree of dysmenorrhea is correlated to amount of flow, duration of flow, and time of menarche.

- Scant flow with symptoms throughout period is consistent with cervical stenosis.
- Primary dysmenorrhea usually starts a few months after menarche when pt becomes ovulatory.

Does the pt have any accompanying symptoms?

Nausea, vomiting, diarrhea, headache, and dizziness can all accompany dysmenorrhea.

- Symptoms should be recorded and tracked during management.

Dyspareunia and a history of infertility suggest endometriosis.

Does pt have a history of pelvic surgery or pelvic infections?

Adhesions and healed areas of inflammation can cause pain during menstruation.

Does the patient have a family history of dysmenorrhea?

Strong family histories can condition an individual's pain response.

What is the pt's current and past social history?

Stress and tension can play a large part in the etiology of dysmenorrhea.

- Pain is usually gradual in onset and generally worse at specific times of stress.

Lack of sleep and caffeine consumption can intensify symptoms.

Is the pt currently using an intrauterine device (IUD)?

The IUD is a potential cause of dysmenorrhea.

Does pt have any medical conditions contraindicating NSAIDs?

NSAIDs play a major role in the management of dysmenorrhea.

- Medical conditions contraindicating their use include:
  - ◆ Ulcers or inflammation of the GI tract
  - ◆ Chronic renal disease
  - ◆ Aspirin allergy (nasal polyps, angioedema, and bronchospasm)

O   Perform pelvic exam

A scarred or disfigured cervix should be probed to make sure os is patent.
Uterosacral ligament nodularity should raise suspicion for endometriosis.
Uterus may contain fibroids.
Adnexal exam may reveal masses.

Does the pt have up-to-date chlamydia and gonococcus cultures?

Pelvic infection can lead to dysmenorrhea symptoms.

- Pts should have cultures obtained if no recent results are available or if history discloses possible exposure.

Consider complementary imaging studies

The following studies may help elicit causes of secondary dysmenorrhea:

- Pelvic ultrasound
  - ◆ Hydrosonography
- Hysterosalpingography
- Hysteroscopy
- Laparoscopy

Dysmenorrhea
Primary dysmenorrhea is pain without organic disease.
  • Typically found in adolescents with onset shortly after menarche.
Secondary dysmenorrhea is pain as a result of organic disease.
  • Typical onset is after age 20 and is associated with some identifiable organic
    disease.
  • The following are causes:
    - Cervical stenosis   - Small ovarian cysts   - IUD
    - Intrauterine adhesions   - Pelvic congestion   - Fibroids
    - Adenomyosis/Endometriosis   - Uterine retroversion   - Polyps

 Primary dysmenorrhea
Treatment is selected depending on pt's current sexual activity status.
  • Sexually active
    ◆ There are two first-line agents.
      • Oral contraceptives
        ◆ Provide contraception and are effective in 90% of patients suffering from
          dysmenorrhea.
      • The progesterone-containing IUD
        ◆ Also effective in treating symptoms.
  • Currently abstinent
    ◆ NSAIDs
      • Ibuprofen 600 mg PO q6h PRN
      • Naproxen 250 PO q6h PRN
    ◆ COX-2 specific inhibitors
      • Valdecoxib 20 mg PO q12h PRN
  • Oral contraceptives or NSAIDs can be added to the primary treatment as needed
    for nonresponders.

Secondary dysmenorrhea
Treatment is focused on underlying etiology.
  • Cervical stenosis
    ◆ Dilation of the cervical os
      • Dilation & curettage
      • Laminaria
  • Endometriosis
    ◆ Medical and surgical managements (see Chronic Pelvic Pain, p. 76)
  • Intrauterine adhesions, fibroids, and polyps
    ◆ Hysteroscopic resection

Consider alternative treatments
Stress reduction and behavioral modification techniques might be useful.

S   **What are pt's future childbearing plans?**
Pts who are interested in long-term contraception should consider hormone
contraception because barrier methods are difficult to use consistently for long
periods.
If pt has an absolute contraindication to pregnancy (coexisting medical condition), a
barrier method should be used in addition to a primary method of contraception.

Is the pt in a new or nonmonogamous relationship at present?
Barrier methods are the preferred contraceptive method for new or nonmonogamous
relationships.

**Does the pt have a history of STDs or pelvic inflammatory disease
(PID)?**
Pts with a history of infection with gonococcus, chlamydia, or PID should use
condoms to prevent recurrence.
Transmission of viral STDs, such as HIV, HPV, and HSV, is decreased with condoms.

Does the pt have a history of toxic shock syndrome (TSS)?
Pts with a history of TSS should avoid barrier methods other than condoms.

Does the pt have an allergy to latex?
Latex allergy may be life-threatening.
Alternative materials such as polyurethane should be used.

Is the pt comfortable with inserting and removing a barrier device?
This is prerequisite to their use.

O   **Physical exam**
An annual well woman exam should be encouraged and updated when prescribing
contraceptive counseling but is not necessarily a prerequisite to using barrier
methods.

A Contraceptive Counseling, Desires Barrier Method

P Prescribe method

Cervical cap

- Requires fitting and spermicide co-use.
- Place < 6 hrs before use.
- Can be used for up to 48 hrs.
- Typical failure rates is 20% to 40%.

Diaphragm

- Requires fitting and spermicide co-use.
- Place < 6 hrs before use.
- Can be used for up to 24 hrs.
- Typical failure rate is 12%.

Condoms

- Types include male condom and female condom.
- Materials include latex, polyurethane, silicone rubber, and lamb skin.
  - ◆ Lamb skin condoms do not protect against STDs.
- Need to apply before genital contact and remove before loss of erection.
- Usually use with spermicide.
  - ◆ Use water-based lubricants (oil-based lubricants can cause condom breakage).
- Typical failure rate is 14% to 20%.

Prescribe emergency contraception

Every pt on a barrier method should be prescribed emergency contraception for use as a backup in case of slippage, breakage, or retention in vagina (see Emergency Contraception p. 84).

S **Has the pt ever used injectable contraception before?**
Pts who have had a good experience previously should do well.
Pts with previous complaints should consider an alternative.

What is the pt's recent menstrual and intercourse history?
If there is a possibility the pt could be pregnant, she will have to wait until this can be ruled out before starting injectable contraception.

Does pt have a history of irregular periods?
Irregular menses needs a workup before starting injectable contraception.

Does the pt have any of the following that might contraindicate using depot medroxyprogesterone acetate (MPA) injectable?
History of depression or other mood disorder
  • Depot MPA may exacerbate depression, anxiety or PMS symptoms
Obesity or concern about weight gain
  • May worsen with depot MPA use.
Liver disease
Breast cancer
Aminoglutethimide use
  • Reduces depot MPA efficacy
Chest pain, cardiovascular disease, myocardial infarction, stroke

Does the pt have a history of gestational diabetes?
Such pts are at increased risk for diabetes if using depot MPA and should select alternative contraception.

What are the pt's future childbearing plans?
Depot MPA use can delay a return to fertility for an average of 10 months after cessation.
  • Should be avoided in pts desiring immediate fertility upon cessation.

Is the pt aware of the non-contraceptive benefits of depot MPA?
Knowledge of the following non-contraceptive benefits increase pt compliance:
  • Decreases menstrual blood loss (reduces risk of anemia)
  • Diminishes dysmenorrhea symptoms (cramps and pain)
  • May improve endometriosis symptoms
  • Reduces risk of PID and ectopic pregnancy
  • Reduces risk of endometrial (and possibly ovarian) cancer

O **Perform pregnancy test depending on recent menstrual and intercourse history**
Pts exempt from pregnancy test include those:
  • Currently on a regular menses
  • Currently using an alternative and reliable method of contraception
  • Practicing abstinence since last period

A **Contraceptive counseling, desires depot MPA**

Depo MPA consists of a depot of 150 mg of medroxyprogesterone acetate and provides 13 weeks of protection

Mechanisms of action:

- Thickens cervical mucus (blocks sperm passage)
- Inhibits LH surge (prevents ovulation)
- Alters tubal motility
- May alter endometrium

P **Start injectable contraception**

If none of the above contraindications are present, start pt on depot MPA.

- Pts can start any time during first 5 days of menses.
- If there is any possibility of current pregnancy, the pt has two choices:
    - Wait until next menses to start.
    - Use a barrier method for 2 wks, establish a negative pregnancy test, and then start.
- First-time users should be monitored for 15 minutes for allergic or vasovagal reaction.

Counsel pt on side effects

Depot MPA can cause weight gain.

Depot MPA can cause mood changes

- Depression
- Anxiety
- Fatigue
- PMS

Depot MPA may cause a hypoestrogenic state, which can lead to:

- Bone loss
    - Encourage pt to take supplemental calcium and vitamin D.
    - Teens should take 1300 mg and adults 1000 mg supplemental calcium daily.
- Hot flashes
- Decreased libido
- Vaginal dryness, dyspareunia

Counsel pt on possible menstrual changes

Users of depot MPA will encounter irregular bleeding that usually decreases over time.

- 50% of women achieve amenorrhea by 1 year.

Schedule next shot

Follow-up depot MPA in 11 to 13 wks

S **What is the pt's recent menstrual and intercourse history?**
Last menstrual period
Previous period
Any prior unprotected intercourse in current cycle?

When was the last act of unprotected intercourse?
Date and time of last unprotected intercourse should be reviewed.
- General rule is to initiate emergency contraception (EC) within 72 hours.
- Can be started after 72 hours; however, works better closer to the time of intercourse.

Has the pt used EC or oral contraceptives before?
Review with pt use and tolerance of any previous EC or oral contraceptives.
- Pt may have a preference for a particular regimen if it was used before and tolerated well.

Does pt have any contraindications to using EC?
History of any of the following contraindicates EC use:
- Undiagnosed abnormal uterine bleeding
- Hypersensitivity to estrogen or progesterone

The following contraindicate estrogen-containing EC:
- Current migraine headache
- History of deep vein thrombosis or pulmonary embolus

Is the pt currently breastfeeding?
Pts who are breastfeeding should use progesterone-only pills.

Will the pt be driving or operating machinery while using the EC?
Antiemetics, traditionally prescribed with EC to minimize the side effect of nausea and vomiting, can cause drowsiness.

O **Consider pregnancy test**
If intercourse history raises suspicion for conception before last intercourse, perform pregnancy test.
- EC will not work as an abortifacient in pts who are already pregnant.

Physical exam
BP and PE is not necessary before prescribing EC.

A   Unprotected intercourse, desires emergency contraception

P   **Educate pt about possible side effects**
Nausea/vomiting
Breast tenderness
Mood changes
Change in timing of next menses
- Early menses if EC taken in 1st half of cycle
- Delayed menses if EC taken in 2nd half of cycle

Prescribe emergency contraception
EC is available in one of two forms:
- Combined (estrogen and progesterone) pills
- Progesterone-only pills

Multiple formulations can be used.
- Selection of regimen is based upon:
  - Practitioner preference/experience
  - Cost
  - Pt preference
  - Availability
    - Not all prepackaged kits are available (see below).
- EC using *combined pills* is available in prepackaged kit, which contains 4 pills.
  - Each pill contains ethinyl estradiol 50 µg and levonorgestrel 0.25 mg.
  - Take 2 pills immediately and 2 pills 12 hrs later.
  - If prepackaged kit is not available, *almost ANY oral contraceptives can be used.*
    - Use multiple pills so that each dose contains at least 100 µg ethinyl estradiol and either 1 mg of norgestrel or .50 mg of levonorgestrel.
    - Take 1 dose immediately and 1 dose 12 hrs later.
- EC using the *progesterone-only pill* is available in a prepackaged kit, which contains 0.75 mg levonorgestrel.
  - Take 1 pill immediately and 1 pill 12 hrs later.

If not using prepackaged kit, show pt *in detail* how to use oral contraceptives.

Prescribe an antiemetic
A long-acting antiemetic should be taken *1 hr before* taking EC.
- Meclizine 25–50 mg PO × 1

Plan regular contraceptive use (see individual Family Planning sections pp. 80–90)
Pills can be resumed immediately after EC use.
- Use 7-day backup (condoms) if new start.
Depot medroxyprogesterone acetate can be given immediately.

Follow-up instructions
Pregnancy test is necessary if menses has not occurred by 3 wks.

S **What is the pt's recent menstrual and intercourse history?**
If there is a possibility the pt is currently pregnant, contraception needs to be withheld until nonpregnant state can be confirmed.
Insertion of intrauterine device (IUD) while on menses is associated with a higher risk of expulsion.

Does the pt have a history of irregular periods?
Abnormal uterine bleeding (AUB) needs a workup before starting intrauterine contraception (see AUB p. 72).

Does the pt have heavy or crampy periods?
The levonoregestrel IUD improves dysmenorrhea and menorrhagia.
The copper IUD may *increase* dysmenorrhea and menorrhagia.

What are the pt's future childbearing plans?
Because of the cost, IUDs are generally used for pts who would like a prolonged (> 2 years) period of contraception.
- Pts wanting to conceive sooner should use an alternative contraceptive method.
- The copper IUD is effective for 10 years.
- The levonoregestrel IUD is effective for 5 years.

Does the pt have multiple partners or a history of pelvic inflammatory disease (PID)?
These pts are generally not considered candidates for IUD use.
- PID during IUD use can lead to a higher chance of infertility.

Does the pt have any complaints of vaginal discharge?
Pts infected with bacterial vaginosis are at increased risk for PID with IUD use.

Are the pt's Pap smear and STD tests up-to-date?
All tests should be confirmed to be normal and up-to-date before IUD use.

Does the pt have any general questions about IUD use?
Several misperceptions exist about IUD use (e.g., mode of action, etc.).

Does the pt have any contraindications to copper usage?
Wilson's disease or allergy to copper contraindicates the copper IUD.

O **Perform "wet mount" for any undiagnosed vaginal discharge**
See Vaginitis p. 114

Perform pregnancy test depending on recent menstrual and intercourse history
Pts exempt from a pregnancy test include those:
- Currently on a regular menses
- Currently using an alternative and reliable method of contraception
- Practicing abstinence since last period

Perform pelvic exam
Cervix
- Inspect for any discharge that might indicate cervicitis.
Uterus
- Verify uterine position.
  - Anterior/mid/posterior
- Assess for any abnormal contour
  - Fibroids can distort the uterine cavity and increase the rate of expulsion.

A **Contraceptive counseling, desires copper IUD**
The copper IUD is a T-shaped polyethylene device with two flexible arms for insertion.
- Each arm is wrapped with sleeves of copper.
- Effects contraception by working as a functional spermicide.
- Effective for 10 years.

Contraceptive counseling, desires levonorgestrel IUD
The levonorgestrel IUD is a T-shaped device that releases 20 μg of levonorgestrel per day.
- Effect on contraception is by thickening cervical mucus, altering uterotubal fluid and sperm migration.
- May prevent implantation and ovulation.
- Effective for 5 years.

P **Counsel pt on risks of insertion**
Uterine perforation
- Increased risk when uterine position is not established before insertion.

Infection
- Usually occurs within first 3 wks after insertion.
- Increased risk with current bacterial vaginosis or active cervical infection.

Vasovagal reaction
- Increased risk with low pain threshold or stenotic os.

Counsel pt on risks of use
Possible failure
- Increased ectopic rate if failure occurs.

Possible tubal damage/infertility
- PID during IUD use increases the risk of tube scarring and secondary infertility.

Counsel pt on possible menstrual changes
Users of the copper IUD will encounter irregular bleeding that usually decreases over first weeks.
- 50% of women achieve amenorrhea by 1 year.

Users of the levonorgestrel IUD may have spotting for up to 6 months.
- 20% of women have amenorrhea at 1 year.

Insert the copper IUD or levonorgestrel IUD

Schedule follow-up
Customary follow-up is made in *1 month* to verify IUD remains in place.

Counsel pt on "warning" signs
Pts with any of the following should return to the clinic immediately:
- Pain, vaginal bleeding: May signal perforation.
- Missed period: May signal pregnancy (failed contraception).
- Fever, chills: May signal infection.
- Missing strings: May signal expulsion or migrating IUD.

S Has the pt ever used the pill before?
Some pts have a specific brand in mind that works well for them.

How did the pill work for pt in past?

What is the pt's last menstrual period and intercourse history?
If there is a possibility the pt could be pregnant, she will have to wait until this can be ruled out before starting oral contraceptives.

Does pt have a history of irregular periods?
Irregular menses needs a workup before starting the pill.

Does the pt smoke?
Smokers over 35 y/o should not use the pill.

Does the pt have any medical problems that might contraindicate using a pill that contains estrogen?

- Uncontrolled hypertension	- Liver disease
- Biliary disease	- Seizures, migraine headaches,
- Uncontrolled diabetes	blurry vision
- Breast cancer	- Blood clots
	- Chest pain, cardiovascular disease

Is the pt currently taking any medications?
Many anticonvulsants and some antibiotics decrease steroid levels in women taking oral contraceptives, rendering them subtherapeutic.
- Exercise caution with concurrent use of the following:

- Barbituates	- Phenytoin
- Carbamazepine	- Felbamate
- Topiramate	- Vigabatrin
- Rifampin	- Griseofulvin

Is the pt currently breastfeeding? If so, for how much longer?
Combined oral contraceptives lower breast milk volume.
- These pts are candidates for the progestin-only pill until they complete breastfeeding.

O Measure blood pressure
Estrogen can exacerbate hypertension.

Perform pregnancy test depending on recent menstrual and intercourse history
Pts exempt from pregnancy test include those:
- Currently on a regular menses
- Currently using an alternative and reliable method of contraception
- Practicing abstinence since their last period

A Contraceptive counseling, desires oral contraceptives

P **Rule out pregnancy**
If there is any possibility of current pregnancy, the pt has two choices:
- Wait until next menses to start pill.
- Use a barrier method for 2 wks and then establish a negative pregnancy test.

Start pt on an oral contraceptive
If none of the above contraindications are present, start pt on an oral contraceptive.
Start date will be based primarily on current day of menstrual cycle and recent
intercourse history and secondarily on pt preference.
- Pts currently on menses can start on any day of the 1st week of cycle (customarily Sunday).
  - Barrier protection should be used for 1 wk.
- Pts who are not currently on menses and not using an alternate method of contraception need to rule out pregnancy first (see above).

Become familiar with a few formulations of varying strengths and choose from these
The following are examples of oral contraceptive formulations:
- Monophasic (the progesterone dose always stays the same)
  - 20 μg ethinyl estradiol/0.1 mg levonorgestrel
  - 30 μg ethinyl estradiol/1.5 mg norethindrone acetate
  - 35 μg ethinyl estradiol/0.4 mg norethindrone
- Triphasic (the progesterone dose changes during the cycle)
  - 35 μg ethinyl estradiol/0.18- 0.215- 0.25 mg norgestimate
- Progestin-only
  - 0.35 mg norethindrone
If a pt has had a good experience previously with a particular formulation, try the same formulation again.
Breastfeeding women and those with contraindications to estrogen should use the progestin-only pill.

Become familiar with common problems regarding missing pills
If pt misses 1 pill:
- Take missed pill immediately and the following pill as scheduled.
If pt misses 2 pills:
- During first half of cycle
  - Take 2 pills/day for next 2 days and use barrier method until menses.
- During third week of cycle (or 3 pills at anytime)
  - Start new cycle and use barrier protection for 1 wk.
Consider emergency contraception (EC)
- An alternative to "making up" for missed pills is to take EC.
  - Especially useful if intercourse has occurred in last 3 to 5 days.
  - If pt uses EC, *skip any missed pills* and resume taking the remaining pills the day after completing EC (see Emergency Contraception p. 84).

S **What are the pt's future childbearing plans?**
Only pts who are certain they have completed childbearing are candidates for
sterilization.

Does the pt know that there are alternatives to sterilization?
Explanation of long-term alternatives and their typical failure rates as compared to
sterilization should be explained to pt.
- IUD
  - Efficacy up to 10 years.
  - Failure rate comparable to tubal sterilization.
- Vasectomy
  - Efficacy and failure rate similar to tubal sterilization.
  - Lower morbidity and mortality compared with tubal sterilization.

Does the pt understand that sterilization is permanent?
Tubal reanastomosis is the surgical repair of fallopian tubes to make them functional
again.
- Although this procedure is available, its *success is highly variable,* and it should
  not be relied on as a way for pts to regain their fertility if they later "change their
  mind."

Does the pt understand the risks of this procedure?
Provide counseling regarding general risks of having a surgery:
- Bleeding
- Infection
- Surgical damage to organs adjacent to fallopian tubes
- Anesthesia risks

Does the pt understand the possibility of failure?
Every sterilization procedure carries a risk of failure (see below).
- The younger the pt is at time of sterilization, the higher the failure rate.
- Tubal sterilization failures have an increased risk of ectopic pregnancy.
  - One-third of failures are associated with ectopic pregnancy.

Does the pt understand that sterilization does not protect against STDs?
Pts should be counseled that sterilization does not protect against STDs and that a
barrier method is required for such protection.

Is the pt's partner in agreement with this method?
Inquiry should be made into partner's views on the procedure.
- Opposition from partner, or conversely, pressure from partner is not uncommon.
- Discordance between partners may affect the relationship after sterilization and
  be a source of pt regret.

How is the pt's relationship in general?
Pts who are likely to regret sterilization have unstable relationships.

O **How old is the pt?**
Sterilization should be avoided in young pts because they tend to have more time in
their reproductive lives to change their minds.

What is the pt's weight?
Obese pts are poor surgical candidates because of technical difficulties associated with
their habitus.

A   Desires permanent sterilization

P   Plan timing of procedure

Pregnancy must be ruled out before procedure.

- A negative pregnancy test is reliable if pt reports a history of abstinence or consistent use of contraception for the preceding 2 wks.

Choose procedure

Sterilization can be performed by three different methods:

- Ligation
  - ◆ Usually performed for postpartum pts.
  - ◆ Involves occlusion of the tubes with suture followed by transection.
  - ◆ A piece of each tube is removed and sent to pathology for identification.
    - Because of removal and identification of a segment of tube, this procedure has lower failure rates than electrocautery or mechanical procedures.
  - ◆ Failure rate = 0.7%
    - Pomeroy technique
      - ◆ Traction on tube upward to form loop, ligation at base and transection
    - The Irving
      - ◆ Segmental resection, proximal end buried in uterus, distal in mesosalpinx
    - The Uchida
      - ◆ Dissection of tube from serosal covering and burying proximal end in mesosalpinx
- Electrocoagulation procedures
  - ◆ Performed for interval procedures (pt not postpartum)
  - ◆ Done through laparoscopy
  - ◆ Failure rate = 1% to 2%
    - Unipolar coagulation
    - Bipolar coagulation
- Mechanical occlusion
  - ◆ Performed for interval procedures (pt not postpartum)
  - ◆ Uses rings and clips to occlude tube
  - ◆ Greater success rates of tubal reanastomosis (if pt regrets sterilization in future)
  - ◆ Failure rate = 1% to 3.5%
    - Silastic ring
    - Spring clip

Counsel pt on long-term follow-up

Sterilization becomes effective immediately.

Because of increased risk of ectopic pregnancy associated with sterilization failures, pt needs to have pregnancy test performed if menses is ever missed.

- If pregnancy test is positive, ectopic must be ruled out.

S **What color is the discharge?**

Lactation is usually clear or white.

Yellow or green discharge should raise suspicion for local breast disease.

Does the pt have any bloody discharge?

This is more suspicious for cancer.

Does the pt have abnormal periods?

Abnormal periods or amenorrhea may represent a hypoestrogenic state that will need to be addressed in management plans.

- One-third of pts with galactorrhea will have normal menses.

Did the pt recently deliver?

In the absence of breastfeeding, galactorrhea beyond 12 months postpartum deserves workup.

Does the pt use any medications or street drugs?

Several phenothiazine-like compounds, antidepressants, antihypertensives, opioids, and amphetamines can induce galactorrhea.

Has the pt had any recent trauma, surgical procedures, or anesthesia?

All of these can lead to increased prolactin secretion.

Does the pt have excessive stress or a history of prolonged suckling?

Both can be the cause of elevated prolactin.

O **Perform a detailed breast exam**

Examine all quadrants of the breast, starting at the base and moving toward the nipple.

- Secretions should be discharged from multiple ducts when a hormone imbalance is the etiology.
- Single-duct discharge is more suspicious for serious pathology.

Does the pt have hirsutism?

Anovulation secondary to hyperprolactinemia can cause hirsutism.

What is the result of the prolactin test?

Blood should be drawn in the morning.

Normal prolactin levels are 1–20 ng/mL.

Prolactin levels > 100 ng/mL require special attention (see radiologic workup).

What is the result of the thyroid-stimulating hormone (TSH) test?

All pts with galactorrhea should have a TSH level checked.

- Hypothyroidism (diagnosed by an elevated TSH) results in increases in thyroid-releasing hormone, which directly stimulates prolactin release from the pituitary.

What are the results of the radiologic workup?

All pts with galactorrhea should have a coned-down view of the sella turcica.

- The primary purpose of this procedure is to rule out a prolactinoma that is large enough to cause anatomic distortion in the cranium.

All pts with an abnormal sella turcica or prolactin > 100 ng/mL should have an MRI evaluation.

- The cutoff value of 100 ng/mL is empiric based on the fact that most large tumors will have values above this level.

Rule out systemic disease with the following:
CBC
Serum chemistries
U/A
- Liver and renal disease can cause elevated prolactin.

 Galactorrhea

All hormonal etiologies of galactorrhea lead back to the final common pathway of *elevated prolactin levels.*

- Most cases of hyperprolactinemia can be attributed to prolactin-secreting adenomas of the anterior pituitary.
  - These tumors are classified into one of two groups based on size:
    - Microadenomas < 10 mm in size
    - Macroadenomas ≥ 10 mm in size
- The differential diagnosis of hyperprolactinemia includes:
  - Medications
  - Trauma
  - Stress
  - Prolonged suckling

P Consider treatment for microadenomas
Treament for a prolactin-secreting microadenoma is not always necessary and is based on:
- Pt's desire for fertility
- Degree of breast discomfort from lactation
- Presence of amenorrhea (hypoestrogenic state)

Start bromocriptine for pts who desire to get pregnant or have a significant breast discomfort from galactorrhea.
- Bromocriptine is a dopamine agonist that binds to the dopamine receptor in the pituitary and blocks the release of prolactin.
  - Starting dose is bromocriptine 2.5 mg PO qd.
  - Increase to 2.5 mg bid as needed.

If pt has amenorrhea (and fertility is not desired and lactation is not a major problem), estrogen replacement in the form of birth control pills can be the sole treatment.
Microadenomas should undergo radiologic surveillance and prolactin levels annually for 2 years.
- If stable, pt can be followed subsequently with annual prolactin levels.

Treat all macroadenomas
Treat all macroadenomas for shrinkage of tumor and maintenance.
- Start with medication.
  - Macroadenomas might require bromocriptine up to 10 mg/day.
    - Monitor prolactin levels for response every 3 months and repeat MRI after 1 year.
  - Surgery for medical nonresponders (tumor extension), very large tumors, persistent visual symptoms, or bromocriptine side effects.
    - Transsphenoidal neurosurgery

S **How long has the pt noticed the hirsutism?**
A rapid onset of symptoms is suspicious for an androgen-secreting tumor.
Polycystic ovary syndrome (PCOS) usually has a gradual onset of hirsutism beginning
  in the late teens or early twenties.

Does the pt have abnormal periods?
Anovulation is strongly associated with hirsutism.
Pts who are anovulatory and hirsute should be tested for insulin resistance.

Is the pt taking any medications or over-the-counter supplements?
    - Phenytoin-Minoxidil   - Cyclosporine   - Diazoxide
    - Exogenous androgens (dehydroepiandrosterone sulfate [DHEAS],
        an androgen, is a popular food supplement)

Does the pt have any signs of hyperandrogenism other than hirsutism?
Other clinical features include acne, increased libido, and virilization.

Family history
Certain ethnic groups and familial patterns are associated with hirsutism (idiopathic
  hirsutism) and adrenal hyperplasia.

Social history
Review lifestyle for possible drugs or environmental factors associated with hirsutism.

Is the pt pregnant?
Luteomas and theca lutein cysts can arise secondary to human chorionic gonadotropin.

Is the pt peripubertal?
These pts are more likely to suffer from nonclassical adrenal hyperplasia.

O **Perform physical exam**
General
- Moon facies and buffalo hump suggest Cushing's syndrome.
- Generalized obesity is associated with PCOS and truncal obesity suggests
  Cushing's syndrome.

Skin
- Note type of hair growth and distribution.
  - Vellus hair is unpigmented and soft whereas terminal hair is dark and coarse.
- Acne
  - Acne is a sign of hyperandrogenism.
- Acanthosis nigricans
  - Darkened areas of skin around axilla, neck, and groin secondary to
    hyperinsulinemia
- Skin signs of Cushing's syndrome
  - Purple abdominal striae, thin and bruised skin

Extremities
- Thin extremities and muscle wasting are associated with Cushing's syndrome.

A **Hirsutism**
Hirsutism can be described as a change from vellus to terminal hairs.
Hirsutism represents a hyperandrogenic state from an underlying metabolic
  abnormality.

There are 3 "compartments" in which androgens are produced, each with a *specific* androgen:
- The ovaries → Testosterone
- The adrenal glands → DHEAS
- The peripheral tissues → 3α-diol G

The differential diagnosis includes:
- Anovulatory, hyperandrogenic state   - Cushing's syndrome
- Idiopathic (familial) hirsutism   - Nonclassical (late-onset)
- Androgen-producing tumor (ovarian or adrenal)   adrenal hyperplasia

P Rule out ovarian and adrenal tumors

The most important part of the hirsute workup is ruling out ovarian and adrenal tumors.

- Tumors originating from the ovary that cause hyperandrogenism can be expected to produce excess testosterone.
  - A total testosterone level > 200 ng/dL raises suspicion for a tumor.
- Androgen-producing tumors originating from the adrenal gland can be expected to have elevated levels of DHEAS.
  - DHEAS > 800 μg/dL indicates adrenal pathology.

Rule out nonclassical (late-onset) adrenal hyperplasia
Measuring a 17α-hydroxyprogesterone level tests for nonclassical adrenal hyperplasia.
- A level < 200 ng/dL rules out the disease.

Rule out Cushing's syndrome
Cushing syndrome should be considered in all hirsute pts and screened for when history and PE suggest the diagnosis.
Screening is performed with an overnight dexamethasone suppression test.
- Dexamethasone 1 mg PO is given at 11 P.M., plasma cortisol is drawn at 8 A.M.
  - Cortisol > 10 μg/dL suggests Cushing's syndrome.
  - Cortisol < 5 μg/dL is normal.

Consider testing for hyperinsulinemia
Pts with anovulation and hirsutism should have insulin resistance checked with a 2-hr glucose tolerance test.

Start low-dose oral contraceptives (primary treatment)
Oral contraceptives treat hirsutism by several mechanisms:
- The progesterone component suppresses LH, which lowers testosterone production.
- The estrogen component induces sex hormone–binding globulin, which increases testosterone binding and decreases free testosterone.

Treatment effects will take at least 6 months to notice.
Old hairs will not be affected and need to be removed mechanically.

Consider adding antiandrogen (secondary treatment)
Spironolactone treats hirsutism by several mechanisms:
- Inhibition of androgen production in the adrenals and ovaries
- Competition for the androgen receptor in the hair follicle and inhibition of 5α-reductase

Finasteride inhibits 5α-reductase activity.

S **What is the pt's age?**
Age is the single most important factor in assessing fertility.

Fertility drops markedly after age 35.

How long has the pt been trying to get pregnant? Is the couple having regular, unprotected intercourse?
Review intercourse history, such as frequency and technique, presence of dyspareunia, possible use of spermicidal lubricants.

Has the pt been previously pregnant? Has the male partner sired any children (without current partner)?
Previous conception by either partner can help focus workup.

Has the pt had any previous workup?
Note previous tests and treatments.

Does the pt or partner have a history of STDs?
STDs place the pt at risk for reproductive organ scarring, which can cause infertility.

Does the pt have normal (monthly) periods?
Regular, monthly periods is the easiest sign to confirm monthly ovulation.
Mittelschmerz (midpain), premenstrual symptoms, and cervical mucus change also suggest ovulation.

Does the pt have a history of gynecologic problems?
History of pelvic pain, prior gynecologic surgery, and intrauterine device use raises suspicion for anatomic abnormalities.

O **Perform physical exam**
General: Hirsutism? (polycystic ovary syndrome) Acanthosis nigricans? (insulin resistance)
Neck: Thyroid (abnormalities are associated with infertility)
Pelvic: Anatomic abnormalities? Pain?

Is there evidence of ovulation?
Ovulation can be inferred or confirmed by the following:
- History of normal menstrual cycles
- Elevated progesterone in midsecretory phase
- Gross evidence of ovulation on U/S

What is the result of the semen analysis?
Normal semen analysis is:

- Volume	2 mL or more
- Concentration	20 million/mL or more
- Motility	40% or more with forward progression
- Morphology	60% or more normal forms

What is the result of the hysterosalpingogram?
A hysterosalpingogram is a radiographic image of the pelvic anatomy.
- Performed by injecting radio-opaque dye into the uterine cavity and tubes.
- Images are assessed for any structural abnormalities (fibroids, polyps, tubal distortion).
- The "spill" of dye from the fallopian tubes into the peritoneal cavity indicates tubal patency.

Consider U/S
U/S can help survey pelvic organs beyond the PE.

Consider hysterosonogram or hysteroscopy
Hysterosonogram is a U/S survey of the uterus after its cavity has been distended with
water (by catheter).
Hysteroscopy involves direct visualization of the uterine cavity and tubal ostia (tube
openings to uterus).

Infertility
Failure to conceive despite regular unprotected intercourse for 1 year
- Primary infertility
  - ◆ No previous pregnancies
- Secondary infertility
  - ◆ At least one previous pregnancy

Etiology
- Anatomic (Tubal or Pelvic)   35%
- Male Factor   35%
- Anovulation   15%
- Unexplained   10%
- Other (including Cervical)   5%

Treat anovulation with ovulatory induction agents
Two main classes of induction agents:
- Clomiphene citrate
  - ◆ Works centrally to antagonize estrogen receptors and "trick" body into
    thinking it is deficient in estrogen.
  - ◆ In response, natural gonadotropins are increased in order to stimulate ovaries
    to produce an egg.
  - ◆ Starting dose is 50 mg (max up to 250 mg) daily on menstrual cycle days 3–7.
- Gonadotropins
  - ◆ Injectable medications that directly stimulate ovaries to produce eggs
  - ◆ Examples include follitropin alpha and follitropin beta

Treat male factor infertility with intrauterine insemination (IUI) or intracytoplasmic sperm injection (ICSI)
IUI uses a catheter to bypass the cervix and introduce sperm directly into the uterine
cavity.
- Indications include oligospermia, antisperm antibodies, and cervical factor.

ICSI has revolutionized the treatment of male factor infertility.
- Performed in laboratory; process of injecting a single sperm into egg

Treat anatomic problems with surgical correction
Surgically correctable defects include fibroids, polyps, and adhesions.
Surgery is performed with hysteroscopy or laporoscopy.

Treat unexplained infertility with in-vitro fertilization (IVF)
Multistep process whereby gametes are retrieved from both partners, egg is fertilized in
laboratory, and embryo is placed directly into uterus.
Eggs are surgically retrieved from the female after heavy stimulation of ovaries with
gonadotropins.

S **When was the pt's last menstrual period?**
This information provides the practitioner with an idea of how long the pt has been in
   menopause and guides treatments.

Is the pt currently experiencing any symptoms?
Hot flashes, day sweats, night sweats
  • Insomnia (secondary to night symptoms)
Decreased libido
Genital dryness
  • Secondary dyspareunia
Urinary incontinence

Does the pt smoke?
Smoking exacerbates the symptoms of menopause and adds to osteoporosis risk.

Does the pt have any risk factors for depression?
Menopause does not cause depression, but women with a history of of depression
   (including postpartum depression and PMS) are susceptible to recurrence during this
   time of physical and emotional stress.

Does the pt have any risk factors for osteoporosis?
Osteoporosis is a leading cause of morbidity for postmenopausal women.
Risk factors include:
  - Smoking   - Menopause without estrogen replacement
  - Low body weight   - Sedentary lifestyle

O **Perform physical exam**
Weight and blood pressure
Breasts
Pelvic
  • External genitalia: Atrophy, signs of inflammation
  • Speculum: Perform PAP smear
  • Bimanual: Abnormalities in uterus, pelvic masses

Consider follicle-stimulating hormone (FSH)
Menopause can be confirmed with FSH > 34 IU/L

Review results of the most recent mammogram
The annual postmenopausal exam provides a good time to review previous
   mammogram; results encourage continued surveillance.

A **Menopause**
12 months of amenorrhea after age 40
Average age is 51 years

P **Provide symptom relief**
Most symptoms of menopause can be relieved with hormone (estrogen) replacement.
In women with an intact uterus, a progesterone must also be given to protect the
  endometrium from unopposed estrogen.
- Examples of combination hormone replacement therapy (HRT):
    - 0.625 mg conjugated equine estrogens/2.5 mg medroxyprogesterone acetate
    - 1 mg estradiol/0.5 mg norethindrone acetate
    - 5 μg ethinyl estradiol/1 mg norethindrone acetate
Provide counseling on short- and long-term use of HRT:
- Much debate in the literature is currently surrounding the use of HRT.
- Appropriate counseling in terms of interpreting the current literature and relative
  risks should be provided to all HRT new-starts.
Other treatments
- Hot flushes: Remove triggers, dress in layers
- Vaginal dryness: Lubricants, moisturizers
- Depression: SSRIs

Provide osteoporosis preventive counseling
Osteoporosis/Fractures
- Nonpharmacologic therapy
  - Weight-bearing exercise   - Fall-prevention counseling
  - Alcohol limits   - Smoking cessation
- Pharmacologic treatments for the prevention of osteoporosis and fractures
    - Bisphosphonates: Alendronate 5–10 mg PO qd or 35–70 mg PO weekly
    - SERMs: Raloxifene 60 mg PO qd
    - Calcitonin: Calcitonin-salmon 1 spray (200 units) in alternating nostrils daily
    - Calcium/Vitamin D
      - Total daily intake of calcium (diet and supplement) should be at least 1500
        mg without HRT and 1000 mg with HRT.
      - Consider Vitamin D supplementation for pts at risk for low levels.
- Consider dual-energy x-ray absorptiometry (DEXA) scan.
    - The DEXA scan is used to diagnose osteopenia and osteoporosis and guide
      treatment and prevention.
    - Results are reported as "a score."
    - A "T score" compares the pt's bone mineral density (BMD) with the mean
      BMD value of a young adult:
      - Normal   Less than –1.0 SD of the young adult mean
      - Osteopenia   Between –1.0 and –2.5
      - Osteoporosis   More than –2.5

S   What is the pt's menstrual history?

Menstrual cycles normally range from 21 to 35 days.

- As menopause approaches, cycles become irregular.
- Large variability between consecutive cycles is common.

Does the pt have a sense that she is entering perimenopause?

Pt perception can be predictive of menopausal onset.

Is the pt experiencing any of the following symptoms of perimenopause?

Hot flashes, night sweats
Vaginal dryness
Urinary incontinence

Is the pt experiencing any sexual dysfunction?

Sexual dysfunction is a common problem among perimenopausal women.

- Symptoms can be secondary to physical or hormonal changes of perimenopause.

Does the pt have a history of depression?

Although perimenopause does not cause depression, women with a history of depression are susceptible to recurrence during this time of physical and emotional stress.

Has the pt had a hysterectomy?

An ovarian-sparing hysterectomy is associated with an earlier menopause secondary to altered ovarian blood flow.

Does the pt smoke?

Smokers experience earlier menopause than nonsmokers and tend to have a shorter transition.

O   What is the pt's age?

Age is one of the most important factors in determining perimenopausal state.
Median age of perimenopause is 46 to 47 y/o.

Perform PE

Weight and blood pressure
Thyroid

- Hypothyroidism is a common disease of women in their forties and can mimic perimenopausal symptoms.
  - Should be screened for in the presence of menstrual irregularities and suspicion on PE.

Breasts
Pelvic

- External genitalia: Atrophy, signs of inflammation
- Speculum: Perform Pap smear
- Bimanual: Abnormalities in uterus, pelvic masses

Is the vaginal pH elevated?

Elevated vaginal pH in the absence of pathogens is associated with a hypoestrogenic state.

Consider follicle-stimulating hormone (FSH) and inhibin B levels

Changes in these hormones may signal perimenopause; however, these hormones can fluctuate markedly.

Perimenopause is associated with elevated FSH (> 24 IU/L) and low inhibin B
(< 30 ng/L).
- Estradiol is highly variable, especially in early perimenopause, where it can
  actually be elevated.

Perimenopause
Time between regular periods and cessation of menses when periods become irregular
in length and often heavier.
- Early perimenopause: Cycle irregularity with < 3 months of amenorrhea
- Late perimenopause: Cycle irregularity with 3 to 11 months of amenorrhea
Average age of onset is 46 years old; average duration is 5 years.

Provide symptom relief
Most symptoms of perimenopause can be relieved with oral contraceptives (OCs).
- OCs regulate periods, relieve vasomotor symptoms or genitourinary atrophy, and
  provide contraception.
- Start with low-dose OC
  - Formulations containing 20 μg of ethinyl estradiol
  - Avoid with smokers (> 15 cigarettes/day)

Consider antidepressants for depressive symptoms

Consider endometrial biopsy (EMB)

All perimenopausal-age pts with irregular bleeding need an EMB.

Provide lifestyle counseling
Perimenopause is the start of a major change in a woman's life and provides an
excellent opportunity for education and promotion of general healthy living.
- Diet
  - Review healthy dietary habits with an emphasis on calcium intake for the
    prevention of osteoporosis.
    - Reproductive-age women should be taking a total of 1000 mg calcium/day.
    - Consider Vitamin D supplementation for pts at risk for low levels.
- Exercise
  - Aerobic exercise promotes a healthy cardiovascular system.
  - Weight-bearing exercise maintains bone health.
- Smoking
  - Contributes to worsening of many perimenopausal issues such as vaginal
    dryness, cardiovascular disease, and osteoporosis.

Offer screening tests
Mammogram
- Every 1 to 2 years beginning at age 40
- Annually after age 50
Cholesterol
- Beginning at age 45, cholesterol testing every 5 years
Diabetes
- Beginning at age 45, fasting glucose every 3 years

S **Obtain a detailed history of complaints**

Premenstrual syndrome (PMS) symptoms can vary widely, including:

- Bloating	- Feeling of weight gain
- Breast discomfort	- Pelvic pain
- Headaches	- Hot flushes
- Irritability	- Depression
- Crying	- Decreased libido
- Fatigue	- Insomnia
- Thirst	- Hunger

Review PMH

It is important to verify that the symptoms are not attributable to any other medical problem.

- All of the following can worsen in the premenstrual period.
  - ♦ Depression
  - ♦ Intestinal problems
  - ♦ Migraines
  - ♦ Arthritis

O **Physical exam**

A compete PE should be performed to rule out any medical problems as the etiology.

A **Premenstrual Syndrome**

A group of symptoms, both physical and behavioral, that occur in the second half of the menstrual cycle

They are followed by a period that is entirely free of symptoms, and they often interfere with work and personal relationships.

- Up to 50% to 75% of women experience some combination of PMS symptoms.

Premenstrual Dysmorphic Disorder

A psychiatric term to diagnose a "severe" form of PMS characterized by a marked interference with daily activities and relationships.

- Only about 5% of pts meet this criteria.

P **Symptom diary**

A symptom diary is the most effective way to manage PMS.

- Symptoms are recorded daily and rated on a severity scale of 1 to 4.
  - ♦ Stress the importance of documentation of the top three to four symptoms that most affect the pt's quality of life.
  - ♦ Document menstrual period days.

Keeping a diary helps target treatments to symptom specifics.

- Documents symptoms over time with patterns and associations.
- Avoids underestimation of symptoms.

Initiate treatment

Medical approaches to therapy

- NSAIDs
  - ♦ Good if principal symptom is cramping, heat intolerance, or diarrhea
  - ♦ Generally very safe
  - ♦ Use intermittently (as needed during symptoms)
- Antianxiety drugs
  - ♦ Benzodiazepines

- ◆ Good for symptoms that predominate around anxiety
- ◆ Not good for long-term use
- Diuretics
  - ◆ Good if main symptom is feeling of bloating or weight gain
- Birth control pills
  - ◆ Efficacy unclear
  - ◆ New progesterone, drospirenone, may be effective
- Gonadotropin-releasing hormone agonists
  - ◆ Dangerous potential for side effects: osteoporosis
- Selective serotonin reuptake inhibitors (SSRIs)
  - ◆ Serotonin plays a role in PMS through an unclear relationship with estrogen.
    - Estrogen appears to promote serotonin production and prevents its degradation.
    - Three regimens to take SSRIs for PMS:
      - ◦ Continuous
      - ◦ Intermittent
        - Taking SSRI only during last 2 wks of cycle
      - ◦ As needed
  - ◆ Side effects include interrupted sleep and sexual dysfunction.

Complementary and alternative medicine
- Nutritional approaches (diet)
- Botanical medicines
- Vitamins
  - ◆ Magnesium: 200–400 mg/day
  - ◆ Vitamin B_6: Can damage nerves > 100 mg/day
  - ◆ Calcium: 1200–1600 mg/day
    - Added benefit of osteoporosis prevention
- Mind-body approaches
  - - Relaxation   - Aerobic exercise
  - - Guided imagery   - Light therapy
  - - Group therapy   - Massage
  - - Yoga

S **Obtain a detailed history of all pregnancies and losses**

The fetal *gestational age* at the time of loss is important to note.

- Etiologies of recurrent loss tend to cluster in groups according to gestational age.
  - Second trimester losses should raise suspicion for anatomic problems.
    - Antiphospholipid syndrome (APS) is associated with losses after 10 wks' gestation.
- Age estimates by last menstrual period are not always accurate because fetal death often occurs "silently" several weeks earlier.
- Age estimates by measuring the fetal size on U/S are more accurate.

Elicit any history of genetic diseases or anomalies

Familial reproductive problems suggest possible genetic etiologies.

Is the pt taking any medications or drugs, smoking or using alcohol, or have any occupational exposures to teratogenic substances?

All of these factors have been associated with early pregnancy loss.

Lead, mercury, solvents, and ionizing radiation are all teratogens.

Has the pt had any previous pelvic infections, uterine instrumentation, or diethylstilbestrol (DES) exposure?

This history can suggest anatomic distortion leading to pregnancy loss.

- Synechiae are scars in the uterine cavity usually secondary to instrumentation.
- DES is a synthetic estrogen used in the 1970s for threatened abortions and has been associated with early pregnancy losses.

Is history compatible with cervical incompetence?

Cervical incompetence follows a classic pattern:

- Painless dilation
- Leakage of fluid (rupture of membranes)
- Delivery of a live fetus

Does the pt have any chronic medical illnesses or galactorrhea?

Uncontrolled diabetes, thyroid disease, and thrombophilias are all associated with recurrent pregnancy loss (RPL).

Hyperprolactinemia is also associated with pregnancy losses.

Any prior workup or treatments?

Note any prior studies and treatments in order to focus the workup.

Karyotyping of previous losses provides important information on possible chromosomal problems.

O **Height, weight, body habitus, and blood pressure**

Perform PE

Breasts
- Galactorrhea

Cervix
- Evidence of trauma
- Malformation

Uterus
- Note size and shape

Does the pt have any signs of diabetes or hyperandrogenism?

Signs of diabetes mellitus (DM) mandate a workup for glucose intolerance.

Acne and hirsutism are signs of hyperandrogenism.

Recurrent Pregnancy Loss

RPL is classically defined as the loss of three first trimester pregnancies or one second
trimester pregnancy.

The cause of RPL is elicited in only 60% of cases.

- Proposed causes of RPL and their incidences are as follows:
  - Genetic (5%)   - Endocrine (17%)
  - Anatomic (12%)   - Autoimmune (50%)
  - Infectious (5%)   - Other (10%)

P **Rule out anatomic etiologies**

Hysterosalpingogram is the gold standard.

- Plain x-ray film of *uterine cavity and tubes* after filling with radioopaque dye

Hydrosonogram

- Instillation of saline into uterine cavity followed by visualization by U/S

Hysteroscope

- Instrumentation used to directly visualize the uterine cavity and tubal ostia

Rule out APS

The two most common laboratory tests to rule out APS (see APS p. 12) are:

- Anticardiolipin antibodies
- Lupus anticoagulant

Obtain karyotype of both partners

Most common abnormality found is balanced translocations:

- Two-thirds reciprocal
- One-third Robertsonian

Consider infectious etiologies

Ureaplasma urealyticum has been associated with RPL.

Consider other endocrine or metabolic disorders

    - TSH   - Prolactin
    - Homocysteine   - Luteal phase defect   - DM

Treat anatomic defects

Treat anatomic defects according to the obstetric history:

- Cervical incompetence
  - Cerclage
- Septated uterus, submucosal myomas, and synechiae
  - Hysteroscopic resection

Treat APS

Daily low-dose aspirin (80 mg)
Subcutaneous heparin 7500 U q12h

Treat chromosomal abnormalities

Preconceptional counseling
Genetic counseling early in pregnancy

Treat endocrine causes

Hyperhomocysteinemia

- Folate

Luteal phase defect

- Progesterone supplementation or empiric clomiphene citrate

S **Is there a possibility the pt is currently pregnant?**
Always consider pregnancy first when pt complains of amenorrhea.

Obtain a detailed menstrual and contraceptive history
Last menstrual period
Previous cycle lengths

Is the pt taking any hormone contraception?
Hormone contraception such as the levonorgestrel IUD or the depot
   medroxyprogesterone acetate injection can cause amenorrhea.

Is the pt currently suffering from any stress?
Emotional or psychological distress can cause hypothalamic dysfunction.

What is the pt's diet?
Dietary restriction can lead to hypothalamic dysfunction.

What are the pt's exercise habits?
Excessive exercise can lead to hypothalamic dysfunction.

Does the pt have a family history of premature menopause?
Review family history for potential genetic inheritance of ovarian failure.

Does the pt have a recent history of uterine curettage?
Asherman's syndrome (uterine synechiae) is more likely after uterine curettage.

O **Check pt's age**
Pts older than 45 should be considered for perimenopause or menopause.

Perform PE
General
   • Obesity (BMI > 30) is associated with excessive cortisol production and
      polycystic ovary syndrome (PCOS)
Skin
   • Check for evidence of hirsutism and acanthosis nigricans, which are seen in
      PCOS.
Pelvic
   • Vaginal atrophy or dryness suggests hypoestrogenic state.

Perform pregnancy test
This is the single most important test in the workup of secondary amenorrhea.

Draw the following labs to assess hormonal status
      - TSH   - Estradiol
      - FSH   - Prolactin

Rule out systemic disease with the following
CBC
Serum chemistries
U/A

A **Secondary Amenorrhea**
Secondary amenorrhea is defined as 6 months without menses or a time equivalent to three of the previous cycle intervals without menses.
- A workup can be initiated upon pt presentation regardless of duration.

A general diagnosis of "secondary amenorrhea" is given to these pts while a workup attempts to find a definitive etiology.
- Most patients will have secondary amenorrhea caused by anovulation.
  - Other possible etiologies include:
    - Asherman's syndrome   - Ovarian failure
    - Prolactin tumors   - Hypothyroidism
    - Excess cortisol   - Excess androgens (PCOS)
    - Hypothalamic suppression caused by stress, diet, or exercise
    - History of using depot medroxyprogesterone acetate

P **Perform progestational challenge test**
Management of secondary amenorrhea consists of a series of tests designed to locate where in the hypothalamic-pituitary-ovarian-uterine axis the dysfunction lies.
The first step is to perform a progestational challenge test.
- This test confirms a functional ovary (capable of making estrogen) and a functional uterus (outflow tract).
- The test is performed by administering medroxyprogesterone acetate 10 mg PO q day for 5 days.
  - If a period results, the uterus and ovaries have been confirmed to be working and a diagnosis of anovulation can be made.

If progestational challenge test is negative, administer estrogen followed by progesterone
Administration of estrogen and progesterone mimics a normal hormonal cycle as produced by a normally functioning hypothalamus, pituitary, and ovary.
- If a period ensues, the problem lies in the ovaries or in the central nervous system.
- If withdrawal bleed is absent, suspect Asherman's syndrome.

If period ensues with estrogen and progesterone, check gonadotropin levels
Gonadotrophs (FSH and LH) are released from the pituitary in response to gonadotropin-releasing hormone released from the hypothalamus.
- Their target organ is the ovary.
  - Therefore, high levels of gonadotrophs indicate an unresponsiveness of the ovary (ovarian failure).
  - Low or normal levels indicate a pituitary or hypothalamic problem.

If gonadotrophs are low, perform a coned-down view of sella turcica
The sella turcica is the cranial bone in which the pituitary lies.
- A pituitary tumor affecting gonadotroph secretion would visibly distort the cranial anatomy on x-ray.
  - A normal x-ray implies that amenorrhea is the result of hypothalamic dysfunction.

The following is a description of an encounter for pts requesting *screening* for STDs. Refer to individual SOAPs (vulvar ulcers, vulvovaginitis, PID) for treatment of *current* infection.

S Assess risk by history

The following categories place women at high risk for STDs:
- Adolescents to 25 years of age
- History of STD
- Multiple partners
- New partner
- Pt exchanges sex for money or drugs.
- Partner or self is current or past user of IV drugs.
- Partner is homosexual or bisexual.

Provide counseling on prevention

Provide information on risk factors (above) and risk reduction:
- Condoms provide best protection.
- Oral contraceptives increase cervical mucus and thus prevent ascending infection (PID) but not lower genital tract infection (cervicitis).
  - Only to be used as an adjuvant to barrier method.

O Perform PE

External genitalia: Inspect for warts, ulcers, and other lesions.

Cervix: Discharge may indicate a cervicitis.

Bimanual: Tenderness in the adnexa may indicate a subclinical salpingitis.

Perform appropriate tests

Cervical swab
- *Chlamydia trachomatis* and *Neisseria gonorrhoeae*
  - Collect sample as endocervical swab.
  - Specimen stored in tube that lyses organisms and detects DNA by probe.
  - Can be performed at the same time as Pap smear.

Serologic tests
- Syphilis
  - Screening with a "nonspecific" test such as venereal disease research laboratory or rapid plasma reagin (see Vulvar Ulcer p. 112)
- Hepatitis B virus (HBV)
  - Initial screen is performed by the detection of antibody to hepatitis B surface antigen.
- Human immunodeficiency virus (HIV)
  - Immunoassay
- Herpes simplex virus (HSV)
  - Type-specific immunoassays can distinguish exposure between HSV-1 and HSV-2.

Wet mount
- Trichomonas
  - Directly visualized flagellate under saline-prepped slide

A STD Screening

P Provide treatment

Chlamydia trachomatis
- Doxycycline 100 mg PO bid × 7 days (Rec)
- Azithromycin 1 g PO × 1 (Alt)

Neisseria gonorrhoeae
- Ceftriaxone 125 mg IM × 1 (Rec)
- Ciprofloxacin 500 mg PO × 1 (Alt)

Syphilis
- Benzathine penicillin G 2.4 million units IM q week × 3

Trichomonas
- Metronidazole 2 g PO × 1 (Rec)
- Metronidazole 500 mg PO BID × 7 days (Alt)

Genital warts
- Patient-administered:
  - Podofilox 0.5% 3 days on/4 days off × 4
  - Imiquod 5% qhs for up to 16 wks
- Provider-administered:
  - Podophyllin resin
  - Cryotherapy
    - Trichloroacetic acid

Referral

HIV
- Counseling and treatment are complex and evolving.
  - HIV is treated with antiretrovirals and protease inhibitors.

Provide counseling

Partner counseling for all positive results

HSV
- Promote condom use for asymptomatic individuals.
- Encourage discussion about prevention and partner testing.

Offer vaccine

HBV vaccine for pts at high risk for STDs who screen negative.

S **Obtain a detailed history**
How many times a day does the pt urinate? (> 8 times/day is considered excessive)
Does she lose urine when coughing, laughing, or sneezing? How often?
Does she have nocturia? How many times a night does she get up?
Does she experience urgency or frequency?
Does she lose urine before "making it to the bathroom"? (symptom of urge
  incontinence)
Does she wear a pad for the incontinence?

Does the pt have pain?
Pain may indicate interstitial cystitis or urinary tract infection (UTI).

**Has the pt had a previous surgery for urinary incontinence? Previous
pharmacologic treatment?**
Pts with previous treatment require more detailed evaluation.
  • A record of prior medicine used can help tailor recommendations.

**Does the pt have glaucoma, gastroesophageal reflux disease, or
dementia?**
These medical problems can be exacerbated by anticholinergics, the drugs of choice in
  treatment of overactive bladder.

Does the pt have diabetes?
Can lead to urinary frequency.
Can be a risk factor for neurogenic bladder (paresis).

Is the pt taking any medicines?
Antihypertensives, cholinergic agents, neuroleptics, and xanthines can all cause
  incontinence.

Is the pt postmenopausal?
Hypoestrogenic states can lead to urogenital atrophy and irritative symptoms.
Urogenital tissue is responsive to replacement estrogen cream.

O **Perform detailed PE**
Urethra: Check pain associated with diverticula.
Bladder
Signs of pelvic floor relaxation (cystocele, rectocele, enterocele)
Evidence of loss of urine under Valsalva (supine, sitting, and standing)

What are the findings on simple cytometric evaluation?
Simple cytometrics are performed as a way of defining the etiology of the problem.
  • Direct visualization of the genitourinary anatomy (urethra and bladder) with a
    cystoscope.
  • Simulation of bladder filling with CO_2 gas or water and observation for signs of
    bladder (detrusor muscle) contractions and bladder capacity (hyperdistention).
  • "The Q-tip test"
    ◆ A cotton-tipped applicator is inserted into urethra
    ◆ The angle the cotton-tipped applicator makes with the floor represents the
      angle of the urethral-vesicular junction (UVJ).
    ◆ Test is considered positive if, under Valsalva pressure, this angle can be
      observed to change > 30 degrees.

What is the result of the U/A and culture?
Always rule out a UTI in the workup of the incontinent pt.

A **Urinary Incontinence**
The two most common diagnoses are:
- Genuine stress urinary incontinence (GSUI, also known as hypermobile urethra)
- Detrusor instability (commonly known as irritable bladder)

Less common etiologies include:
- Overflow incontinence   - Interstitial cystitits
- Neurogenic bladder   - Intrinsic sphincter deficiency

P **DI is treated with pharmacologic agents and behavioral modifications**
Common pharmacologic agents are:
- Anticholinergics and antispasmodics
  - Work by blocking muscaranic activity, thereby avoiding bladder stimulation.
  - Counsel pts on common side effects such as xerostomia and blurry vision.
    - Propantheline 15 mg PO bid
    - Oxybutynin hydrochloride 5 mg PO tid/Oxybutynin ER 5–10 mg PO qd
    - Tolterodine tartrate 1–2 mg PO bid/Tolterodine tartrate ER 4 mg qd
- Adrenergics
  - Work by relaxing detrusor muscle with β-adrenergic stimulation and stimulating the urethral sphincter via α-adrenergic receptors
    - Imipramine 25 mg PO tid
    - Amitriptyline 50 mg PO tid

Behavioral modifications include:
- Maintaining normal amounts of fluid intake during day (5 to 6 glasses of water)
- Avoiding fluid intake at night
- Avoiding alcohol and caffeinated beverages, which increase urine production
- Bladder "training"
  - This involves gradually increasing the time interval between voiding episodes in hopes of establishing a new higher threshold at which urge incontinence occurs.
- Kegel exercises
  - Contraction and relaxation of the pubococcygeal muscles

GSUI is treated with surgery
More than 300 procedures for GSUI have been described.
Gold standard is the retropubic urethropexy:
- Involves "restoring" the UVJ to its original angle.
- Sutures are placed in tissues surrounding the UVJ and used to pull it up and anchor it.
  - Burch procedure: UVJ anchored to ileopectineal (Cooper's) ligament.
  - Marshall-Marchetti-Krantz: UVJ anchored to pubic symphysis.

S Obtain a detailed sexual history

Enquire about any new partners and timing of relations.

- Chancroid (caused by *Haemophilus ducreyi*) and primary herpes simplex virus (HSV) have incubation periods of days to a few wks.
- Primary syphilis has an incubation period of 2 to 4 wks.

Where is the ulcer and when was it first noticed?

HSV recurrence tends to be on the same side of the body.

Is the ulcer new or recurrent, solitary or multiple, and painful or painless?

HSV ulcers can recur often and are markedly painful.

A solitary lesion is likely to be primary syphilis.

- Multiple lesions include HSV and chancroid.

The primary chancre of syphilis is painless.

Does pt have any constitutional complaints or inguinal soreness?

Primary HSV infection is commonly associated with headaches, fever, malaise, and bilateral lymphadenopathy.

Unilateral adenopathy is associated with chancroid.

Does the pt have any abnormal bleeding?

Intermenstrual spotting and cervicitis affect most women with primary HSV infection.

O Note location, depth, number, and consistency of any lesions

HSV infection has multiple superficial lesions that are painful.

Primary syphilis has a solitary, hard, and painless lesion.

Chancroid consists of multiple lesions that may coalesce, are soft and tender, are deep, and have undermined edges with irregular contour.

Perform testing for syphilis

Because untreated syphilis can lead to the serious sequelae of tertiary and congenital infection, all pts with a vulvar ulcer should undergo testing for syphilis.

- Dark-field microsopy is the preferred testing method for primary syphilis but is not readily available in most centers.
- Serologic testing is a good screening method but picks up only 70% of pts at the time of primary chancre.
  - Serologic testing usually begins with a nonspecific "nontreponemal" test called rapid plasma reagin (*RPR*).
  - This test evaluates for the presence of antibodies that react to antigen from beef heart.
  - Results are expressed in titers, and levels usually correlate with disease activity.
    - RPR becomes nonreactive after treatment.
  - A reactive RPR is usually followed by a specific "treponemal" test called *FTA-ABS*.
  - This test evaluates for the presence of specific treponemal antibodies and is reported as positive or negative.
    - A positive result remains reactive indefinitely.

If suspected, perform testing for HSV

Cell culture (only sensitive in currently active lesions)

HSV type-specific serologic assays

Antigen-detection tests (only in active lesions)

If suspected, perform testing for chancroid
Culture for *Haemophilus ducreyi* on selective media

A **Herpes Simplex Virus**
Primary syphilis
Chancroid
Differential diagnosis includes:

- Aphthous ulcers
- Pyoderma gangrenosum
- Granuloma inguinale
- Behçet's syndrome
- Carcinoma
- Lymphogranuloma venereum

P **HSV is treated with one of three antiviral agents: acyclovir, famciclovir, or valacyclovir**
Primary infection can be treated with:
- Acyclovir 400 mg PO tid × 7 to 10 days
- Famciclovir 250 mg PO tid × 7 to 10 days
- Valacyclovir 1 g PO bid × 7 to 10 days

Recurrent infection can be treated with:
- Acyclovir 400 mg PO tid × 5 days
- Famciclovir 125 mg PO bid × 5 days
- Valacyclovir 1 g PO qd × 5 days

Suppressive therapy can be treated with:
- Acyclovir 400 mg PO bid
- Famciclovir 250 mg PO bid
- Valacyclovir 500 mg PO qd

Additional relief can be gained by the following:
- Wash lesions twice daily.
- Take sitz baths.
- Apply warm compresses.
- Wear loose clothing.
- Use local anesthetics.
- Apply cornstarch on panties.

Primary syphilis is treated with:
Benzathine penicillin G 2.4 million units IM × 1

Chancroid is treated with:
Erythromycin 500 mg PO qid × 7 days (Rec)
Azithromycin 1 g PO × 1 (Alt)

Perform HIV testing on all pts suspected of having an STD as the etiology of their vulvar ulcers.

S **Obtain a detailed history of the current complaint**

Discharge

- Duration
- Consistency
- Factors related to onset
- Color
- Previous over-the-counter treatments

Pruritus

Odor

- Pts with bacterial vaginosis (BV) may experience an increase in odor after sexual intercourse secondary to semen-triggered release of amines from anaerobic bacteria.

Does the pt give a history of anything that could upset the normal vaginal environment?

- Any recent antibiotic use?
- Douches?
- Changes of partners?
- Foreign body/tampon use?
- Hormone/contraceptive use?
- Increase in sexual intercourse?

Is the complaint limited to the vulva?

Symptoms limited to only the external genitalia should prompt an allergy review:

- Deodorant soaps?
- Laundry detergents?
- Perfumed or dyed toilet paper?
- Swimming pool chemicals?
- Synthetic clothing?

O **Perform PE**

External genitalia

- Inspect for any of the following:
  - Erythema
  - Edema
  - Ulcers
  - Pallor
  - Excoriations
  - Blisters

Vagina

- Inspect for any discharge:
  - *Candida* is curdy, white, cottage cheese–like.
  - Bacterial vaginosis is thin, dark, and homogenous.
  - *Trichomonas* is yellow-gray or green and frothy.
- Test vaginal pH
  - Test vaginal pH by touching nitrizine paper to the lateral wall of the vagina.
  - Vaginal pH is normally acidic (pH = 3.8 to 4.2) secondary to the predominant flora, lactobacillus.
  - An alkaline pH (> 4.5), as indicated by the paper turning dark blue, is abnormal and consistent with BV or trichomonas vaginitis.

Perform wet mount and "whiff test"

Collect a specimen of discharge with a cotton-tipped applicator and place into 1–2 cc normal saline (NS) in a test tube.

Perform wet prep by placing a drop of NS onto one-half of a microscope slide and a drop of 10% potassium hydroxide (KOH) onto the other side.

- To each of these, add a drop of the vaginal discharge prep.
- Examine NS side for clue cells (consistent with BV) and trichomonads (flagellated protozoa).
  - Presence of many leukocytes in this prep is also consistent with trichomoniasis.
- Examine KOH side for hyphae (evidence of yeast).

Perform "whiff test" by adding a drop of KOH to the vaginal discharge.

- Release of a strong, fishy odor (amines) can be appreciated in the presence of BV and *Trichomonas* infection.

Consider a gram stain and culture

Consider culture for a yeast infection that has failed over-the-counter or prior medical treatment.

Culture is also more sensitive than wet mount for diagnosis of *Trichomonas*.

Gram stain is more useful for BV because culture is not specific.

 Vulvovaginitis

Most causes of vulvovaginitis are infectious.

The three major etiologies are:

- Candida vulvovaginitis
- Bacterial vaginosis
- Trichomonas vaginitis

Less common causes are noninfectious:

- Irritant/chemical
- Atrophic
- Dermatitis
    - Contact, seborrheic, atopic
- Dermatoses
    - Lichen simplex, lichen sclerosus
- Systemic dermatoses
    - Eczema, psoriasis

P **Treat vulvovaginal candidiasis with antifungals**

Numerous intravaginal preparations are available:

- Miconazole 2% cream 5 mg intravaginally for 7 days
- Terconazole 0.8% cream 5 g intravaginally for 3 days
- Clotrimazole 500-mg vaginal tablet for one dose

One available oral treatment:

- Fluconazole 150 mg PO × 1

Treat bacterial vaginosis with metronidazole

Metronidazole gel 0.75%, 5 g per vagina qd for 5 days (Rec)

Metronidazole 500 mg PO bid for 7 days (Rec)

Metronidazole 2 g PO in a single dose (Alt)

- Avoid alcohol while taking medication.
    - Metronidazole can give a disulfiram-like reaction.

Treat trichomonas vaginitis with metronidazole

Metronidazole 2 g PO in a single dose (Rec)

Metronidazole 500 mg PO bid for 7 days (Alt)

- Only *oral* metronidazole is effective against *Trichomonas*.
- *Trichomonas* is considered a sexually transmitted disease.
    - Arrange for treatment of the pt's partner.

V

Emergency Room and Consultations

S Obtain a detailed menstrual history

Describe onset and duration of bleeding.

Number of pads used and degree of saturation (heavy, medium, or light)

Are there any associated cramps?

The answer to this question can help differentiate between threatened and complete abortion; cramping is often felt as the products of conception (POC) are passed through the uterus in a complete abortion.

Intense pain should always raise suspicion for a possible ectopic pregnancy.

O Review VS

Check for signs of cardiovascular instability.

Check CBC

Elevated WBCs may indicate infection; low hematocrit may reflect a hemoperitoneum.

Check β-hCG level

This level is important in interpreting U/S findings.

Check Rh status

All pts with first trimester bleeding should have their Rh D status checked

- Administer 50 μg anti-D immune globulin to pts with Rh D–negative blood.

Perform pelvic exam

Is the cervical os open or closed?

- An open os is consistent with inevitable abortion.
- A closed os is consistent with threatened or complete abortion.

Is there active bleeding?

Is there any POC visible inside the os that can be manually removed?

What is the size and position of uterus?

- This information may be important if surgical therapy is required.

Any adnexal tenderness or masses?

Always consider the possibility of an ectopic pregnancy.

Obtain U/S

U/S directly surveys the contents of the uterus.

- The first embryonic structure to develop that is identifiable by U/S is the gestational sac, followed by the yolk sac, and, finally, the fetal pole.
  - Abdominal U/S is able to detect a gestational sac when the β-hCG level is > 6000 IU/L.
  - Transvaginal U/S is able to detect a gestational sac when the β-hCG level is > 1000–1500 IU/L.

  - The absence of a gestational sac in the presence of β-hCG levels above these cutoff values means that the pt has either a completed abortion or an ectopic pregnancy.

- The following findings on U/S support a diagnosis of inevitable or missed abortion:
  - Collapsed gestational sac
  - Absence of yolk sac when the gestational sac is 8 mm
  - Absence of fetal pole when the gestational sac is 16–18 mm
  - Absence of cardiac motion when embryo is 4–5 mm in length

A **Spontaneous Abortion**

This is a general diagnosis that can be further specified as follows:

- Blighted ovum (aka anembryonic gestation)
  - A gestational sac is > 17–18 mm without an embryo visualized.
- Complete abortion
  - Spontaneous and complete expulsion of all POC from uterus
  - Diagnosis supported by closed os, history of cramping, and an endometrial thickness < 15 mm.
- Incomplete abortion
  - Partial expulsion of all POC from uterus
  - Endometrial thickness > 15 mm and/or continued active bleeding
- Inevitable abortion
  - Cervical dilation and uterine bleeding before expulsion of POC
- Missed abortion
  - Fetal death before 20 wks of pregnancy without expulsion of POC
- Septic abortion
  - Intrauterine infection accompanying abortion

P **Therapeutic options for abortion include surgical, medical, and expectant management**

Treatment choice depends on:

- Condition of pt at time of assessment
- Pt preference

Surgical management

- Dilation and curettage (D&C)
  - Requires an operating room
- Manual vacuum aspiration (MVA)
  - Can be done in the ER or clinic

Medical management

- Vaginal delivery of 800 µg misoprostol (dose may be repeated once in 24 hrs as needed) and waiting up to 2 to 3 days

Complete Abortion

No intervention necessary

Incomplete Abortion

D&C or MVA

Inevitable Abortion

D&C, MVA, or expectant management

Missed Abortion

D&C, misoprostol, or expectant management

Septic Abortion

IV antibiotics

D&C after antibiotics are on-board

S **Obtain a detailed menstrual history**

When was the pt's last menstrual period?

Has there been any irregular bleeding?

- Bleeding associated with ectopic is generally less than with abortion.

Obtain a detailed description of the pain

Characteristic of the pain

- Pain before rupture is usually colicky or vague; after rupture, pain intensifies.

Where is the pain located?

- Site of pain usually corresponds to ectopic site but can be bilateral.
- Shoulder pain can represent diaphragmatic irritation seen with hemoperitoneum.

Assess pt's desire to maintain future fertility

Future childbearing plans often are taken into account when making treatment decisions in the management of ectopic pregnancy.

O **Check VS first**

Check for signs of cardiovascular instability (hypotension and tachycardia).

Consider orthostatics.

Perform abdominal and pelvic exam

Are there signs of peritonitis?

Adnexal tenderness or masses present?

Be careful not to rupture ectopic by applying too much pressure.

Check CBC

Hematocrit will give you an idea of the pt's stability.

Check β-hCG level

β-hCG level, along with U/S, forms the basis of management decisions.

Check Rh status

Rh-negative pts with negative antibody screen need anti-D immune globulin before discharge.

Obtain U/S

Attempts to directly visualize the earliest evidence of a pregnancy: the gestational sac (GS).

- Based on the principle that when the β-hCG level reaches a certain point, the GS should be able to be visualized (in the uterus) by U/S.
- This level is called the "discriminatory level."
  - ✦ Abdominal U/S is able to detect a GS when the β-hCG level is > 6000 IU/L.
  - ✦ Transvaginal ultrasound is able to detect a GS when the β-hCG level is > 1500 IU/L.
- If the β-hCG level is above these "discriminatory levels," and a pregnancy cannot be visualized, a diagnosis of "an abnormal pregnancy" can be made.
  - ✦ If the clinical assessment is highly suspicious for ectopic, the pregnancy can be treated as such.

An ectopic pregnancy can often be *directly visualized* by U/S.

- Findings range from a complex or cystic adnexal mass to visualization of an actual embryo.

Free fluid on U/S is suggestive of hemoperitoneum.

A **Ectopic pregnancy**
The differential diagnosis includes:

- Abortion
- Ruptured corpus luteum
- Dysfunctional uterine bleeding
- Endometriosis
- Salpingitis
- Appendicitis
- Adnexal torsion
- Degenerating fibroid

P **Observation for unclear clinical picture**
If the pt's condition worsens, surgical exploration is necessary.
If the pt's condition remains stable, perform serial CBCs, abdominal exams, and, in 48 hrs, a repeat β-hCG.
- If β-hCG level is not doubled, the diagnosis can be specified as an *abnormal pregnancy* and managed as an ectopic if the clinical picture matches.

Surgical management
The following clinical scenarios mandate surgical exploration:
- Unstable pts
- Pts with ruptured ectopics
- Pts who have completed childbearing
- Pts with contraindications to medical management (see below)

Immediate surgical exploration after stabilization
- Two large-bore IVs, copious fluids, type and cross-match blood, arrange for operative management via laparotomy

Medical management (methotrexate)
Medical management may be considered for pts who are stable and desire future fertility.
- Contraindications to usage include:
  - Hemodynamic instability
  - Mass > 3.5 cm
  - Noncompliant pt
  - Thrombocytopenia
  - Peptic ulcer
  - Fetal cardiac activity
  - β-hCG level is > 6500
  - Elevated liver function tests
  - Renal insufficiency
  - Pulmonary disease

Dosing is 50 mg/m^2 based on body surface area.
Close follow-up of declining β-hCG levels is necessary.
- Check β-hCG level on Day 4 and Day 7.
  - β-hCG level should decline by 15% between Days 4 and 7.
    - If level declines, follow with β-hCG levels q wk.
    - If not, repeat methotrexate or perform surgery.

Follow-up all pts after treatment until β-hCG is negative!

S   **Obtain detailed history of complaint**

Nature of pain
- Hollow organs such as bowel or fallopian tubes are associated with crampy pain.
- Ovarian etiologies are associated with constant, sharp pain.

Location of pain
- Unilateral, lower quadrant pain is suspicious for adnexal problem.
- Bilateral lower quadrant pain can be pelvic inflammatory disease (PID).
- Gynecologic etiologies may present with symptoms and signs referred to the upper quadrants.

Is there bleeding present?

Cramping associated with vaginal bleeding raises suspicion for spontaneous or inevitable abortion or ectopic pregnancy.

Is nausea and vomiting (N/V) present?

N/V is associated with adnexal torsion.

Does the pt have any risk factors for infectious process?

Recent gynecologic procedures

Review PMH

Reproductive-age or postmenopausal women may have history of a medical problem (diverticulitis, PUD) that might focus the workup.

O   **Age**

Prepubertal or adolescent pts have a higher incidence of ovarian torsion.

Vital signs

Verify that pt is stable.
Presence of fever raises suspicion for infectious process.

Perform PE

Pelvic
- Abdomen
  - Rebound, tenderness
  - Bowel sounds
  - Distention
- Cervix
  - Discharge
  - Cervical motion tenderness
- Uterus
  - Enlargement: Associated with fibroids
  - Tenderness: Associated with endometritis
- Adnexa
  - Tenderness
  - Masses
- Rectal
  - Information complements bimanual exam.

Acute Pelvic Pain
The differential diagnosis can be divided into gynecologic and nongynecologic.
Problems of gynecologic origin can further be classified according to pregnancy status:
- Gynecologic—Pregnancy-related
  - Ectopic
  - Abortion
- Nongynecologic
  - Appendicitis
  - Bowel obstruction
  - Pancreatitis
  - GU infections
  - Diverticulitis
- Gynecologic—Nonpregnancy-related
  - Cervicitis
  - Torsion
  - PID (including tubo-ovarian abscess)
  - Degenerating fibroid
  - Endometritis

Perform pregnancy test
A pregnancy test is the single most important evaluation in the workup of acute pelvic pain.

A positive test dramatically focuses the differential diagnosis and places ectopic pregnancy at the top of the list.

Obtain other laboratories:
CBC
- Elevated WBCs can indicate an infectious process.

Comprehensive metabolic panel
- Hepatic or biliary abnormalities may focus the differential diagnosis.

Amylase/lipase
- Consider with pancreatitis.

Consider imaging studies
Imaging studies may complement the PE in narrowing the diagnosis.
- U/S
  - Gold standard imaging test of the pelvic viscera
  - Able to assess organ size, masses, and free fluid.
  - May be able to directly visualize ectopic pregnancy.
- CT
  - Useful when etiology can not clearly be distinguished between abdominal and pelvic origin
- MRI
  - Generally not used in the acute gynecologic setting, but may have a role in the presence of acute pain with a normal pregnancy.

S
What is the pt's menstrual history?
Molar pts usually present with painless vaginal bleeding following a missed menses.
  • Pt may report passage of grape-like vessicles.
Most pts are considered to be pregnant at time of bleeding presentation.

Does the pt have any recent obstetrical history?
Partial moles frequently have been given antecedent diagnosis of missed or incomplete
  abortion.
Some gestational trophoblastic diseases (GTDs) can occur after a term pregnancy.

Does the pt have any excessive nausea or vomiting?
Molar pregnancies frequently have nausea and vomiting symptoms.

Does the pt have any symptoms of hyperthyroidism?
The high hCG level associated with molar pregnancy can stimulate thyroid hormone
  production, leading to hyperthyroidism.

O
Check VS first
Cardiovascular instability (hypotension and tachycardia)
  • Emboli from the molar tissue can occur.
Elevated blood pressure
  • Early preeclampsia (< 20 wks) has been associated with GTD.

Perform PE
Cervix may be open and expulsing hydropic villi.
Uterus may be larger than dates in some complete moles (50%).
Ovaries can be enlarged secondary to hormonal stimulation.

Check CBC
Massive bleeding can occur with moles.

Check β-hCG level
β-hCG level is frequently highly elevated.
  • β-hCG can be > 1 million IU/L with complete molar pregnancies.

  • In normal pregnancy, β-hCG peaks at 100,000 IU/L at about 10 wks.

Thyroid-stimulating hormone (TSH)
High levels of β-hCG can cause stimulation of thyroid gland and symptoms of
  hyperthyroidism.

  • β-hCG and TSH are similar hormones that share the same "alpha subunit."

Check Rh status
Rh-negative pts with no antibodies require anti-D immune globulin before discharge.

What are the results of the U/S?
Complete molar pregnancies are often diagnosed before treatment.
  • The classic appearance of a complete mole is a "snowstorm" pattern on U/S.
U/S may also pick up theca lutein cysts, which result from high levels of β-hCG.

  • β-hCG and luteinizing hormone (LH) are similar hormones that share the
    same "alpha subunit."

What is the result of the CXR?
A CXR should be performed to look for metastatic disease or trophoblastic emboli.

A **Gestational Trophoblastic Disease**

Benign GTD
- Molar pregnancies can be qualified as *complete* moles or *partial* moles.
  - A complete mole results from the fertilization of an *empty egg* by a single sperm, resulting in a haploid set of chromosomes.
    - Complete moles are more common in general and more frequently present with enlarged uteri, very high β-hCG levels (and its systemic sequelae as described above), and a clear diagnosis on U/S.
  - A partial mole results from the fertilization of a normal, haploid egg with *two sperm*, resulting in a triploid pregnancy.
    - A partial mole is a pathologic diagnosis made after examining tissue retrieved from a missed or incomplete abortion.

Malignant GTD
- Invasive mole
- Choriocarcinoma
- Placental site trophoblastic tumor

P **Dilation and evacuation**

Mainstay of treatment of molar pregnancy is evacuation of the uterine contents.
- Cervix must be dilated.
- Suction is followed by sharp curettage and oxytocin administration.
- Blood products must be available because these pts can have massive intraoperative hemorrhage.
- Laparotomy must be prepared for in case a hysterotomy is needed to control bleeding.

Long-term follow-up

All molar pregnancies have the potential to transform into malignant disease (see below).

This can occur as a delay from time of treatment.

Therefore, all pts need to be followed for a period of 1 year with negative β-hCG determinations.
- Start with β-hCG every 1 to 2 wks until negative twice, then monthly for 6 to 12 months.
- Pts with a slow fall in β-hCG should be followed for 2 years.
- Perform physical exams every 2 wks until β-hCG is negative and then every 3 months.

Prescribe contraception during the follow-up period.
- Oral contraceptives are customary.

Evaluate for malignant GTD

Pts with any of the following need evaluation for malignant GTD:
- Metastatic disease (positive findings on CXR)
- Choriocarcinoma
- β-hCG > 20,000 IU/L more than 4 wks after initial treatment
- β-hCG increases at any point in surveillance
- β-hCG plateaus over 3 wks
- Persistently detectable β-hCG 4 to 6 months after evacuation

Treat malignant GTD

A variety of single and multiagent chemotherapy regimens are available.

S **What symptoms is the pt experiencing?**

Symptoms for pelvic inflammatory disease (PID) vary widely from none to severe peritonitis.

Abdominal pain is the most consistent complaint.

Right upper quadrant complaints may signal Fitz-Hugh-Curtis syndrome (PID with perihepatic involvement).

What is the timing of complaints?

Duration of symptoms is usually short (< 2 wks).

Pain secondary to *N. gonorrhoeae* infection has acute onset during or just after menses.

Is the pt at high risk for STDS?

The following are considered high-risk factors:

- Prior history of STD	- Prior PID
- New partner	- Multiple partners
- Symptomatic partner	- Young age
- No contraception	

Does pt have a history of recent instrumentation?

Any procedure that breaks the mucus plug of the cervix increases the chances of ascending infection:

- Endometrial biopsy	- D&C
- Intrauterine device placement	- Hysteroscopy

Does pt appear reliable and compliant?

Consideration of pt compliance should be made when prescribing outpatient therapy (see below).

O **What is the pt's age?**

Younger pts have a higher risk for PID.

Obtain VS

Fever is sometimes present but not necessary for the diagnosis.

Perform PE

Cervix: Assess for presence of mucopurulent discharge and cervical motion tenderness (CMT).

Uterus: Assess for presence of tenderness.

Adnexa: Assess for tenderness and masses.

Rule out ectopic pregnancy

Obtain pregnancy test.

What is the result of the CBC?

WBCs may be elevated but not consistently.

Obtain cultures and consider gram stain

Cultures
- Obtain cultures for *C. trachomatis* and *N. gonorrhoeae*.

Gram stain
- May be useful in the presence of gross cervical pus.
- Perform saline prep of the discharge.
  - Presence of many WBCs suggests PID.

A   **Pelvic Inflammatory Disease**

Diagnosis must be met by the presence of ALL of the following (and absence of another diagnosis):

- Lower abdominal pain and tenderness
- Adnexal tenderness
- CMT

With one additional sign indicating the presence of infection:

- Fever > 38.3° C
- Cervical mucopurulent discharge
- Elevated erythrocyte sedimentation rate
- Elevated C-reactive protein
- Documented infection with *C. trachomatis* or *N. gonorrhoeae*

Most likely pathogens are *N. gonorrhoeae*, *C. trachomatis*, anaerobes, gram-negative facultative bacteria, and streptococci.

P   **Assess severity of disease**

Pts with PID can be treated as outpatients or inpatients.

- Certain criteria have been put forth to guide practitioners in making this decision.
  - The following clinical scenarios mandate inpatient treatment:
    - Pt noncompliance
    - Fever > 38° C
    - Uncertain diagnosis
    - Oral treatment failure
    - Suspected tubo-ovarian abscess
    - Pregnancy
    - Nausea and vomiting (unable to take oral meds)

Start antibiotics

Outpatient

- Recommended
  - Ofloxacin 400 mg PO bid × 14 days **and**
  - Metronidazole 500 mg PO bid × 14 days
- Alternative
  - Ceftriaxone 250 mg IM × 1 **and**
  - Doxycycline 100 mg PO bid × 14 days

Inpatient

- Recommended
  - Cefotetan 2 g q12h **and**
  - Doxycycline 100 mg IV q12h
- Alternative
  - Clindamycin 900 mg IV q8h **and**
  - Gentamicin load 2 mg/kg then 1.5 mg/kg q8h

Monitor response

IV antibiotics can be stopped 24 hrs after clinical response.

Complete a 14-day course of treatment with PO antibiotics (Doxycycline 100 mg bid).

Treat or refer partner

S **Obtain complete gynecologic history**
Include all past infections, operations, and diagnoses.

Is the pt experiencing symptoms because of the mass?
Torsion should be considered in the presence of pain and requires emergent surgery.
Functional cysts do not usually cause pain.
GI symptoms should prompt evaluation of colon.

How long has the mass been diagnosed?
Any mass that is unresolved for more than one cycle needs surgical evaluation.
A simple, cystic mobile unilateral mass that is < 8 cm in a reproductive-age woman can be followed for 6 to 8 wks.

Family history
Inquire about possible hereditary ovarian cancer.

O **What is the pt's age?**
Age is the single most important factor for predicting possible malignancy.
Any size adnexal mass in the premenarche or postmenopausal age group needs surgical evaluation.

Perform PE
Abdomen
- Palpate for any masses.
- Advanced-stage ovarian cancer can produce a rigid abdomen.
  - This is a result of massive tumor infiltration of the omentum, making it a solid organ (a.k.a. "omental caking").
Pelvic (Have pt empty bladder and rectum before exam.)
- External genitalia: Inspect and palpate for any evidence of a mass externally.
- Vault: Inspect and palpate for a mass.
- Cervix: Inspect the cervix grossly for any lesions.
- Corpus
  - Palpate during bimanual exam.
  - Note uterine size, contour, tenderness, and mobility.
- Adnexa
  - Note mass.
  - Describe size (in cm), contour, consistency, and mobility.
- Rectal
  - A rectovaginal exam provides the best information about the nature of any adnexal mass.
  - It is a mandatory part of any evaluation.

Obtain CBC
Elevated WBCs focuses the workup on an infectious etiology such as tubo-ovarian abscess (TOA).

A

Pelvic Mass
Gynecologic etiologies
- Uterus
  - Fibroids
Nongynecologic etiologies
- Bowel
  - Abscess, irritable bowel disorder, CA
- Tubes
  - Salpingitis, paraovarian cyst, CA
- Retroperitoneal
  - Lymphoma
- Ovaries
  - Non-neoplastic
    - Functional cyst, theca lutein cyst, endometrioma, TOA
  - Neoplastic
    - Mature teratoma (dermoid), cystadenoma, fibroma, CA

P

Rule out ectopic pregnancy
Ectopic pregnancy is a common cause of an adnexal mass in the reproductive age.

Obtain U/S to complement PE
U/S is the gold standard test in evaluation of the pt with a pelvic mass.
The following findings on U/S of an adnexal mass raise suspicion for ovarian CA:

- Solid components	- Presence of ascites
- Internal papillations	- Bilateral cysts

Order CA125
CA125 is a tumor-associated surface antigen.
- It is found on most nonmucinous epithelial ovarian cancers but can also be found in association with many benign conditions.
- For this reason, it is not used as a screening test, but should be obtained in the presence of a pelvic mass.

Consider further radiologic studies for evaluation
CT can help evaluate masses in the retroperitoneal area.
Barium enema or colonoscopy can help distinguish a GI lesion.

Observation for masses < 8 cm in the reproductive-age pt
Use of oral contraceptives is thought to speed resolution of functional cysts.
- Persistence beyond 6 to 8 wks mandates surgical evaluation.

Surgical exploration of all suspicious masses in the reproductive-age pt
This includes:
- Mass > 10 cm
- Presence of ascites
- Presence of internal papillations or solid component on U/S

Surgical exploration of all masses in the premanarche or postmenopausal pt
Because these age groups do not have functioning ovaries, all masses are suspicious for CA.

VI

Gynecology Ward

S **How is the pt feeling?**

An initial open-ended question such as this allows the pt to bring up any problems of concern to her.

Is analgesia adequate?

Pain thresholds vary widely among individuals.

- On POD 1, some pts may be able to switch to PO analgesia; some may require additional time on the patient-controlled analgesia or injectable narcotics.

Review surgery with pt

If the pt is awake and coherent, this is a good time to discuss with pt the intraoperative course and findings.

O **Review VS**

Mild fever is common in the 1st 24 hrs postop.

- Usually of no clinical significance

Cardiovascular stability should be confirmed by BP and heart rate.

Document all I/O.

- Urine output should be > 30 cc/hr.

Perform PE

General

- Document general appearance of pt.

Heart

Lungs

Abdomen

- Check for distention.
  - ◆ Fullness that is firm is suspicious for intra-abdominal bleed.
  - ◆ Distention that is tympanic is suspicious for ileus or obstruction.
- Auscultate for bowel sounds.
  - ◆ Usually faint on POD 1
  - ◆ High-pitched sounds may indicate bowel obstruction.
  - ◆ Complete absence may indicate ileus, and diet should be *started cautiously.*
- Inspect wound to verify that it is:
  - ◆ Dry
  - ◆ Clean
  - ◆ Intact
    - Bandage may be removed after 12 to 24 hrs postop.

Genitalia

- Remove vaginal pack if this was placed at the time of surgery (vaginal hysterectomy).

Extremities

- Ensure that antithrombotic devices are in place while pt is confined to bed.
  - ◆ These work by reducing hemostasis by applying pressure to veins
    - Graduated compression stockings
    - Pneumatic compression devices

A **POD I status-post total abdominal hysterectomy—Recovering well**

> Here it is a good idea to write out the procedure performed for easy identification by practitioners who view your note.

P **Start diet**

If no concern about postoperative complications, begin a clear liquid diet.

Advancement of diet to soft and then regular is usually made as bowel function returns.

- Bowel function can be confirmed by the passage of flatus or auscultation of bowel sounds.

Restart medications

For pts with medical problems, medications can generally be restarted on POD 1.

- Examples include medications for hypertension, thyroid disease, or diabetes.

Discontinue Foley catheter

Depending on procedure type, the Foley catheter is usually removed on the 1st postoperative day.

For the first 12 hrs following removal, monitor I/O.

- Replace Foley catheter if pt has trouble or inability to void.
- Urine output < 30 cc/hr is suspicious for ongoing or impending retention.

Assess analgesia

Depending on pt's pain threshold, PO analgesics may be able to be started on POD 1.

Common regimens include:

- Tylenol #3 2 tabs PO q 4–6 hrs PRN pain
- Vicodin 2 tabs PO q 4–6 hrs PRN pain

If pain is significant, it is acceptable to leave IM or IV analgesia in place.

Ambulate

All pts should be instructed to ambulate on POD 1.

- Difficult pts may require the assistance of a physical therapist.

Encourage incentive spirometry

Incentive spirometry prevents and treats atelectasis.

Review CBC

Hemoglobin should reflect intraoperative estimated blood loss.

Elevated WBCs can be a result of surgery itself.

Consider imaging study

Pts with suspicion for intra-abdominal bleed should have radiographic assessment for hemoperitoneum.

- Abdominal and pelvic CT is the study of choice.

Pts with tympanic distention should be considered for evaluation of bowel obstruction.

- Kidneys-Ureters-Bladder x-ray is the study of choice.

S Has pt ambulated?
By the second postoperative day, pt should be out of bed and ambulating.
- Consider analgesia problems (inadequacy or too much) as a reason for the pt to stay in bed.

Is analgesia adequate?
Most pts should be controlled on PO narcotics by this point.
- A minority of pts may still require parenteral analgesics.

Has the pt eaten?
PO intake and appetite gives you an idea of the return of GI function.

Has the pt passed gas?
This is another indicator that the bowel function is returning.
- Pts who pass flatus should be able to be advanced to a regular diet if not previously done.
- Pts who feel "bloated" may benefit from medical therapy:
  - Simethicone 80 mg PO qid

O Review VS
Fever at this point is pathologic and requires a workup.
Ensure that pt is voiding (without catheter) and has maintained adequate urine output (> 30 cc/hr).

Perform PE
General
- Document general appearance of pt.

Heart

Lungs

Abdomen
- Check for distention.
- Auscultate for bowel sounds.
  - Usually regular by POD 2
  - Persistence of absent or decreased bowel sounds is suspicious for ileus.
    - Caution with advancement of diet
- Inspect wound to verify that it is:
  - Dry
  - Clean
  - Intact

Extremities
- Ensure that antithrombotic devices are in place if pt is not ambulating regularly.

Check any outstanding labs
Hemoglobin should be noted (if not previously done).

A POD 2 status-post total abdominal hysterectomy—Recovering well

P **Advance diet**
Advance pt to regular diet (if not previously done).

Tailor analgesia
Most pts should have pain controlled with PO analgesia by POD 2.
Consider changing medication from one PO regimen to another if control is
  inadequate.
  • Options include:
    ◆ Tylenol #3 2 tabs PO q 4–6 hrs PRN pain
    ◆ Vicodin 2 tabs PO q 4–6 hrs PRN pain
    ◆ Motrin 600 mg PO q 6 hrs PRN pain

Continue ambulation and incentive spirometry

Consider infectious workup
Pts with fever (T > 100.4° F) more than 24 hrs after procedure require workup for
  sepsis.
Differential diagnosis for postoperative fever includes:
  - Wound infection   - Infected vaginal cuff hematoma
  - Vaginal cuff abscess   - Ovarian abscess
  - Septic vein thrombophlebitis   - Osteomyelitis pubis
  - Urinary tract infection/Pyelonephritis
  - Upper respiratory infection (URI)/Pneumonia
Start workup with comprehensive PE
  • HEENT
    ◆ Evaluate for URI → Throat exudates, nasal congestion
  • Lungs
    ◆ Evaluate for pneumonia → Decreased breath sounds, rhonchi
  • Abdomen
    ◆ Evaluate for appendicitis/cholecystitis → Rebound, guarding, Murphy's sign
    ◆ Evaluate for wound infection → Skin color changes, wound discharge
  • Back
    ◆ Evaluate for pyelonephritis → Costovertebral angle tenderness
  • Vagina
    ◆ Evaluate for cuff hematoma or abscess → Tender cuff mass, purulent drainage
  • Extremities
    ◆ Evaluate for DVT → Swelling, color changes, Homans' sign
Obtain blood cultures
  • Draw at time of fever for maximum yield.
Consider imaging studies
  • CXR for suspected pneumonia
  • Abdominal CT for suspected abdominal process
Start antibiotics
  • For identified etiology, start appropriate antibiotics.
  • For unclear etiology, start empiric broad-spectrum antibiotics.
    ◆ Gentamicin 1.5 mg/kg IV q8h
    ◆ Clindamycin 900 mg PO q8h

S **Discuss discharge planning with pt**

Depending on the individual's recovery, some pts might be interested in being discharged home on POD 3.

Discharge on POD 4 is also acceptable.

Is analgesia adequate?

Make sure the current analgesics are effective for pt.

Does pt have any last questions about surgery?

After a period of recovery, pts may remember questions they were interested in asking.

O **Review VS**

Ensure that pt remains afebrile and VS are stable.

Perform PE

Heart

Lungs

- Verify absence of crackles (atelectasis).

Abdomen

- Verify that any distention from ileus is resolved.

Wound

- Verify that wound remains clean, dry, and intact.
    - Staples (if used) can be removed on POD 3 or 4.

Extremities

A **POD 3 status-post total abdominal hysterectomy—Stable for discharge**

P **Discharge home**

Pts who are stable may be discharged home on POD 3 or 4.

Prescribe PO analgesia

Prescribe the same analgesics that have been effective while pt has been in the hospital.

- Tylenol 1–2 tabs PO q 4–6 hrs PRN pain

Consider prescribing stool softeners and hormone replacement therapy (HRT)

Postoperative state can induce constipation.

- Docusate sodium 100 mg PO bid

For pts who had their ovaries removed, consider HRT.

Oophorectomy causes a sudden loss of estrogen (normally made by the ovaries).

- HRT will replace estrogen and help prevent menopausal symptoms.
- Recent controversy regarding HRT surrounds usage in *postmenopausal* women.
    - HRT is still generally regarded as safe for *surgically induced menopause.*

Schedule follow-up appointment

Pts are generally seen in 1 to 2 wks for a wound check.

Index